BEFORE THE FIRST BREATH

The Womb's Imprint on the Rising Sign and Personality

**Foreword written by
Lynn Koiner LPMAFA**

CYNTHIA RENEÉ SUMPTER

Dedication

For my granddaughter, Kelis ArmeriD'ior Smith, Leo Rising—golden, lion-hearted, and born to shine. Before your first breath, the Sun was already kissing your crown, teaching you to walk with warmth, courage, and joy. May your roar always be love, your light a beacon, and your presence a blessing wherever you go. This book is a love letter to the radiance that announced you to the world, long before you spoke a word.

Love, Grandma-ma

Contents

Foreword   iv

Introduction   vi

Chapter 1   Aries Rising: The Spark of New Beginnings in the Womb   **1**

Chapter 2   Taurus Rising: Grounding the Gestational Experience   **14**

Chapter 3   Gemini Rising: Embracing Movement and Mental Stimulation in the Womb   **28**

Chapter 4   Cancer Rising: Nurturing and Emotional Currents in the Womb   **40**

Chapter 5   Leo Rising: Radiant Warmth and Self-Expression from the Womb   **54**

Chapter 6   Leo Rising: Radiant Warmth and Self-Expression from the Womb   **67**

Contents

Chapter 7   Libra Rising: Seeking Harmony and Balance from the Womb   **80**

Chapter 8   Scorpio Rising: Intensity, Transformation, and the Womb's Deep Emotions   **92**

Chapter 9   Sagittarius Rising: Expansive Optimism and the Gestational Call to Adventure   **105**

Chapter 10   Capricorn Rising: Enduring Determination and the Weight of Responsibility in the Womb   **118**

Chapter 11   Aquarius Rising: Rebellion, Independence, and the Womb's Urge for Freedom   **129**

Chapter 12   Pisces Rising: Empathy, Creativity, and the Womb's "Tuned-Out" Vibration   **141**

References   **153**

Forward

Over the years, Cynthia Sumpter has taken my six professional courses on medical astrology for certification. The individuals who take my courses are never referred to as "students" since they are all professionals in other holistic health fields. As with Cynthia, they are all professionals seeking to expand their knowledge of astrology.

I am always pleased when anyone, taking my courses, is able to use what they have learned and expand that knowledge into information that is strictly their own intellectual innovation. I applaud original thinking and this is a subject – The Medical Astrological Imprint of Gestation – that has not been addressed before.

My article on the *"Ascendant and the Gestation Period"* was not very long but here Cynthia has expanded on that information into a text that is unique, original, instructive and enlightening. I love her writing style – it is a style that I wish to duplicate in my own books. Her information is direct, to-the-point, easy to read and there is little, if any, filler.

Foreword

This makes her book an excellent reference text for other astrologers. As a reference book, one can easily find the information that is sought, rather than weeding through filler paragraphs. Furthermore, the use of bullets tells me that the author is not going to waste my time. I hope you, as the reader, will enjoy this book as much as I did...

—*Lynn Koiner LPMAFA since 1968*

Introduction

It is often said in astrology that our Ascendant (or Rising Sign) represents our outer demeanor, the lens through which we first meet the world. Many astrologers consider the Rising Sign to be rooted in early childhood conditioning, family background, and the environment we experience as we develop. Yet in her pioneering work, medical astrologer Lynn Koiner suggests that this environmental imprint begins even sooner, specifically, in the prenatal period, during a mother's pregnancy.

According to this theory, the mother's emotional climate, physical health, and day-to-day experiences create a potent "environmental field" in which the fetus is immersed. When the mother feels energetic and enthusiastic, or conversely stressed and overwhelmed, the unborn child absorbs these subtle signals. Over time, this imprint can form the basis of the child's Ascendant traits. For instance, if the mother experiences significant mood swings or embraces a wave of creativity during pregnancy, the child's eventual Rising Sign might reflect the emotional tenor of that gestational journey.

Introduction

Gestation and Medical Astrology
In medical astrology, each sign of the zodiac correlates with particular body systems, health vulnerabilities, and psychological patterns. By connecting these associations with specific stories of maternal experiences, we can see a fascinating overlap:

Physical Conditions: Certain Rising Signs frequently appear when the mother undergoes characteristic health trends (e.g., morning sickness for Cancer Rising, restless energy for Aries Rising, or the mother's extremely health-conscious habits for Virgo Rising).

Emotional Influences: The mother's emotional states, whether characterized by confidence, fear, excitement, or ambivalence, provide a continuous feedback loop for the developing fetus.

Prenatal Shaping of Personality: Through stress hormones, nutrient flows, and nuanced maternal-fetal bonding, the child "learns" particular coping styles or worldviews even before birth.

Introduction

Modern scientific research in prenatal psychology echoes these observations.

Studies show that elevated maternal stress, nutritional factors, and even daily routines can affect a child's stress regulation, temperament, and overall resilience. Thus, although astrology employs symbolic language, it aligns with the broader premise that the prenatal environment contributes significantly to personality formation.

A Journey Through Each Rising Sign
This book explores how the 12 Rising Signs, from Aries to Pisces, can be understood as reflections of the mother's experiences in pregnancy. Each chapter outlines:

Traditional Medical Astrology Associations: The body systems, health considerations, and behavioral patterns linked with each Rising Sign.

Prenatal Themes: Drawing on Lynn Koiner's research, personal anecdotes, and case studies, each sign's hallmark maternal experiences are recounted ranging,

Introduction

rom the surge of independence with Aries to the nurturing immersion of Cancer and the dreamlike detachment of Pisces.

Scientific Parallels: Where possible, modern findings on fetal development, maternal stress, epigenetics, and immune responses give real-world context to how gestational events might contribute to the personality traits that astrology ascribes to the Ascendant.

Practical Guidance: Each chapter concludes with insights on how to navigate the innate physical, emotional, and spiritual tendencies of that Ascendant, offering suggestions for both caregivers and individuals looking to harmonize their nature with conscious self-care.

How to Use This Book
Whether you're an astrologer, a curious parent, or someone intrigued by the mind-body-spirit connection, this book offers a comprehensive lens on prenatal influences and the Ascendant. You might choose to:

Introduction

Explore Your Own Ascendant: Reflect on how your parents described your mother's pregnancy, noting if there are resonances between her emotional environment and your Rising Sign traits.

Study a Loved One's Chart: Friends, partners, or children with the same Rising Sign may share similar prenatal narratives. Use the chapters as a conversation starter, weaving in family stories about how pregnancy unfolded.

Provide Holistic Guidance: For practitioners in holistic health, therapy, or birth support, consider these chapters a unique tool for understanding and discussing the profound interplay between gestation, emerging personality, and later health patterns.

Embracing the Gestational Imprint

Ultimately, the Rising Sign can be seen as the archetypal "mask" or "outer shell" that protects the more vulnerable aspects of the self (represented by the Sun, Moon, and other planetary placements).

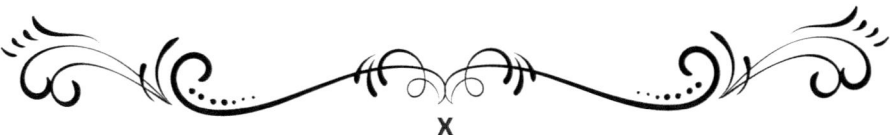

Introduction

By acknowledging that this "mask" may be shaped during the **most formative stage of life, gestation**, we open new avenues for self-awareness and empathy. We can better appreciate why certain individuals enter the world with heightened caution, optimism, or emotional sensitivity.

Far from suggesting our personalities are unchangeably dictated by the womb, these chapters highlight the possibility of understanding, healing, and evolving beyond any limiting imprints. Just as a mother's emotional climate can initially mold the fetus, conscious self-reflection and supportive relationships can modify and enrich our expression of the Ascendant later in life.

By blending astrological wisdom with medical and psychological perspectives, this book celebrates the marvel that we are not solely products of birth but also participants in an ever-evolving journey, guided by the cosmic tapestry that begins to weave itself well before our first breath.

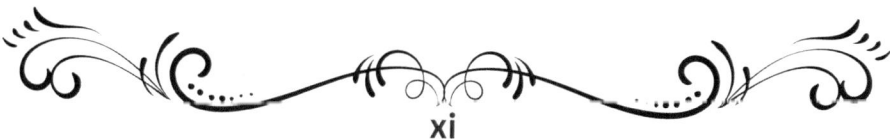

Chapter 1

Aries Rising: The Spark of New Beginnings in the Womb

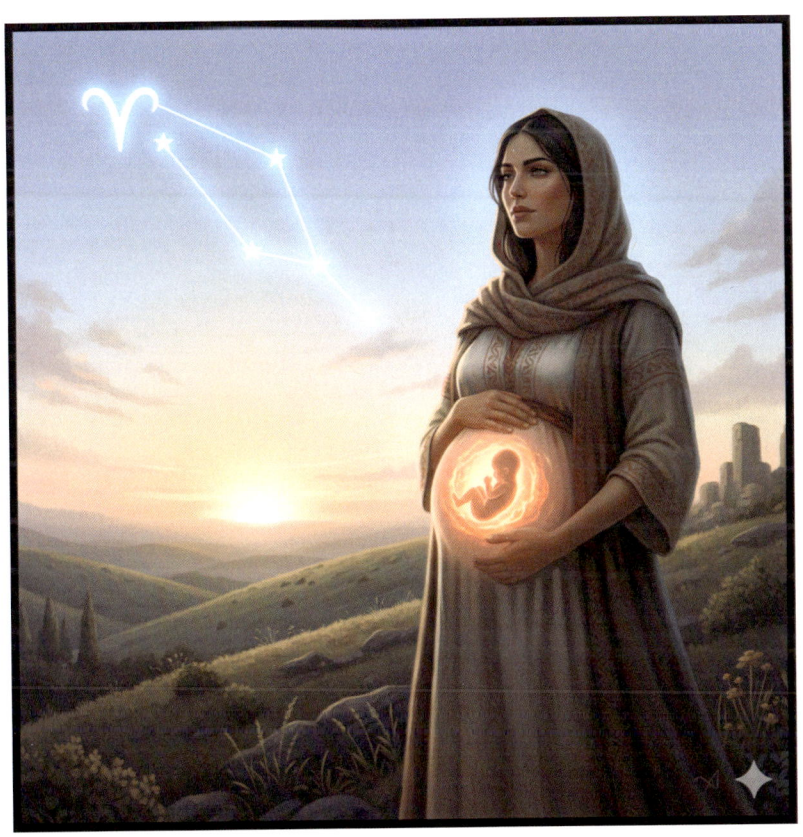

Introduction

Aries is the first sign of the zodiac, a Fire sign ruled by the planet Mars, traditionally associated with courage, initiative, and a pioneering spirit. When a child is born with Aries on the Ascendant (the rising sign), these qualities often translate into a bold, action-oriented approach to life, alongside a passionate readiness to face challenges.

However, as medical astrologer Lynn Koiner suggests, the Ascendant is influenced not only by the birth moment and early environment but also by the mother's attitude, feelings, and experiences during the gestation period. In other words, the "spark" we see in Aries Rising may begin in utero, shaped by maternal emotional, physical, and psychological conditions. Modern prenatal research adds another layer to this perspective by demonstrating how maternal stress, hormone levels, and overall health can have lasting effects on the developing fetus. Aries Rising thus provides a fascinating case study of how astrological tradition and contemporary science can intersect.

Aries Rising in Traditional Medical Astrology

In classical astrology, Aries Rising individuals are described as having:

A"hot"constitution: energetically driven, spontaneous, and prone to short bursts of intense activity.

Physical correlations with the head and upper body: possible susceptibility to headaches, migraines, sinus issues, or inflammation in the face and scalp.

An active "fight-or-flight" response: quick to react to stress, easily aroused to excitement or anger, but also quick to recover.

These traits mirror the planet Mars' energetic symbolism, Mars rules the muscles, adrenals, and blood, all of which tie in closely with an individual's vital force and stress reactivity. Aries Rising people often exhibit high vitality as children, bouncing back rapidly from minor illnesses or injuries. The flip side is a tendency to overexert themselves and, at times, to become headstrong or susceptible to fevers, rashes, and inflammatory ailments,

when under undue stress.

Gestational Theory: The Mother's Role in Shaping Aries Rising

In her work on **gestation and the Rising Sign**, Lynn Koiner proposes that the prenatal environment lays the groundwork for a child's Ascendant traits. Based on interviews and anecdotal evidence, she finds that mothers of Aries Rising children often describe:

Periods of Dynamic Change: Many mothers discovered new hobbies, engaged in fresh pursuits, or underwent significant lifestyle shifts during pregnancy. Some felt a surge of personal growth or an "opening of a new world," echoing the Aries spirit of new beginnings.

Taking Charge Under Stress: Aries thrives on challenge. Likewise, pregnant mothers recalled crises they faced mostly on their own, handling moves, legal battles, or family tensions independently. During gestation, they felt compelled to "do it all" or "take charge," modeling the self-reliance that Aries Rising kids later express.

Impatience and Urgency: Mars is linked with impulse and speed. Aries Rising mothers frequently reported elevated impatience or an intense drive to get things done quickly. The unborn child may absorb this energetic rhythm, emerging with a lifelong tendency to tackle problems head-on.

Feeling Physically Good or Strong: Fire-sign Ascendants (Aries, Leo, Sagittarius) often correlate with mothers who felt robust and positive throughout pregnancy. This "fiery buoyancy" may have biological underpinnings in moderate, well-managed maternal stress (eustress) rather than chronic distress.

By the time the child is born, these gestational imprints may set the tone for a personality that embraces excitement, reacts swiftly to problems, and sometimes chafes at restrictions. The "spark" of Aries Rising can be seen as an echo of the mother's high-energy, crisis-facing pregnancy environment.

Modern Prenatal Research: Linking Biology and Behavior

From a scientific standpoint, there is growing evidence that the womb is a powerful shaper of temperament. Maternal experiences, whether emotional, physical, or environmental, can alter the fetus's developing neuroendocrine and immune systems. The following findings illustrate possible mechanisms by which Aries Rising traits might have biological correlates:

Stress Hormones (Cortisol & Adrenaline):

Chronic or heightened maternal stress during pregnancy elevates cortisol levels, which can cross the placenta and influence the fetus's HPA (hypothalamic-pituitary-adrenal) axis. Children exposed to higher prenatal stress often show increased impulsivity, faster stress reactivity, and a tendency toward more "fiery" or intense responses.

If the mother's stress is episodic and well-managed, rather than overwhelming, it can help the fetus develop resilience, which may account for the Aries Rising child's,

capacity to handle crises with courage.

Inflammation:

Pregnancy-related inflammation (for example, from infection or high maternal C-reactive protein) is linked to neurodevelopmental shifts in the fetus. Some children exposed to excessive inflammation display hyperactive or impulsive traits, patterns reminiscent of Aries' energetic, head-first style.

Aries' "hot" quality resonates with inflammatory physiology: fevers, skin eruptions, and acute infections may align with an inflammatory imprint from the womb.

Prenatal Androgens (Testosterone):

Elevated maternal androgens or heightened fetal testosterone sensitivity can lead to increased assertiveness, competitiveness, and risk-taking in children, traits that echo Aries' "warrior" archetype.

Mars' rulership of Aries often symbolizes masculine or yang energy; modern research on prenatal testosterone,

provides a possible biomedical parallel.

Brain Development and Temperament:

The fetus's limbic system (responsible for emotions) and frontal cortex (executive functions) are shaped by the hormones, nutrients, and stressors in the womb. An Aries Rising child may, therefore, have a heightened capacity for quick, sometimes impulsive decisions, correlating with changes in the development of these brain regions.

Together, these scientific insights support the idea that maternal stress, hormone levels, and emotional states can "program" a fetus for a more active, impulsive, and stress-reactive disposition, matching the classical descriptions of Aries Rising in astrological literature.

Aries Rising in Adulthood: Health and Emotional Patterns

Because Aries Rising is linked with a high-energy constitution, many individuals grow into dynamic adults who:

Seek Action and Novelty: They tend to thrive in environments that offer variety, challenges, and opportunities to lead or innovate.

Exhibit Short-Lived Flare-Ups: Anger or frustration arises quickly, often as a reflex. Yet it also tends to dissipate quickly, like a match that ignites fast and then dies down.

Experience Inflammatory or Stress-Related Issues: Overwork, unmanaged stress, or chronic anger can predispose them to migraines, fevers, skin rashes, or even hypertension if they don't learn healthy coping strategies.

Demonstrate Remarkable Resilience: Aries Rising individuals can rebound swiftly from setbacks or illnesses, thanks to their innate sense of vigor.

Emotionally, they often crave independence and "room to move," reflecting their earliest prenatal experiences of the mother forging ahead on her own terms.

In relationships, they might need partners or friends who respect their drive and give them space to initiate. Learning to channel impatience into constructive action, rather than impulsive outbursts, can be a key developmental task.

Practical Guidance for Aries Rising Natives and Caregivers

Channel the Fire:
Engage in regular physical outlets, sports, dance, cardio workouts, to keep restless energy moving. This helps prevent frustration from building up internally.

Incorporate cooling foods and herbs (e.g., cucumber, mint, chamomile tea) to balance the body's "heat" in times of stress or high activity.

Mindful Stress Management:
Practice breathing exercises, meditation, or yoga to modulate the stress response. Aries Rising can benefit from learning to pause before reacting.

Identify early signs of burnout or inflammatory flare-ups (such as rashes or persistent headaches) and address them immediately with rest and self-care.

Promote Healthy Assertion, Not Aggression:
Support children (and adults) in expressing anger or frustration verbally and constructively. Aries Rising's natural assertiveness can become a strength when harnessed through communication, rather than physical or impulsive outlets.

In family or therapy contexts, understanding that intense outbursts may reflect an underlying sense of urgency helps tailor interventions that channel passion into creativity.

Reinforce Self-Worth:
Many Aries Rising individuals were "gestationally primed" to believe they must handle challenges alone. Reminding them that help is available, and that seeking it doesn't undermine their independence, can foster emotional well-being.

Integrate Prenatal Awareness:

For expectant mothers or future parents, remembering that baby in the womb can absorb not just nutrients but emotional and energetic patterns highlights the importance of stress-management and meaningful support during pregnancy.

Aries Rising or not, a positive, stable prenatal environment promotes resilience and healthier coping strategies for the child.

Conclusion

Aries Rising offers a prime illustration of how **gestational influences, astrological symbolism, and modern science** can converge in our understanding of personality and health. Lynn Koiner's theory that the Rising Sign originates in the mother's emotional and physical environment during pregnancy gains support from current research on prenatal stress, inflammation, and hormone exposure.

The Aries Rising individual, molded in a womb environment brimming with activity, independence, or mild crises, emerges with a fiery and courageous spirit.

Such a child may be predisposed to quick-reacting tempers or inflammatory ailments, yet simultaneously endowed with resilience and an adventurous outlook. Recognizing these formative influences, and addressing them through a balanced lifestyle, emotional awareness, and supportive relationships, can help Aries Rising natives maximize their pioneering strengths while mitigating stress-related vulnerabilities. Ultimately, the story of Aries Rising underscores the profound impact that the mother's body and psyche have on the next generation, even before the first breath is drawn.

Chapter 2

Taurus Rising: Grounding the Gestational Experience

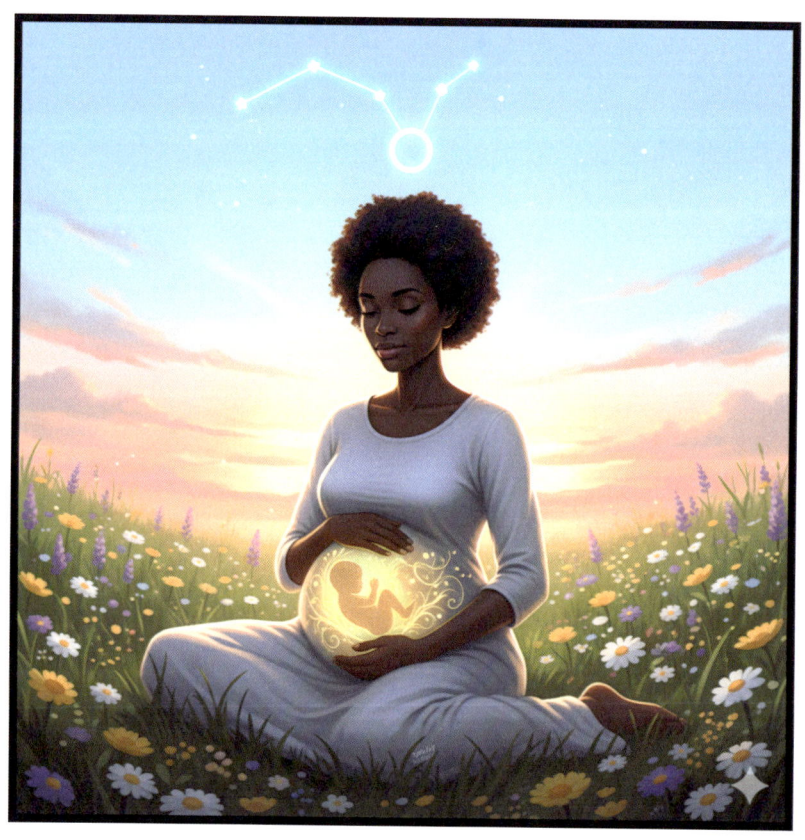

Introduction

Taurus is the second sign of the zodiac, often connected with stability, practicality, and a desire for comfort. Ruled by Venus, Taurus Rising individuals are said to embody serenity, sensuality, and a grounded approach to life. Yet, as with all Rising Signs, Taurus can also reflect a very specific gestational environment experienced by the mother. Medical astrologer Lynn Koiner posits that the incoming child absorbs maternal attitudes and circumstances during the prenatal period; these influences later emerge as the Ascendant traits.

Modern scientific research supports the notion that an expectant mother's psychological, hormonal, and environmental conditions can set foundational patterns in a child's behavior and health. With Taurus Rising, the prenatal atmosphere is often characterized by an emphasis on comfort, creative exposure, and "settling down", qualities that align closely with this sign's earthy, enduring nature.

Taurus Rising in Traditional Medical Astrology

Taurus Rising in Traditional Medical Astrology

Classical texts associate Taurus with the throat, neck, and thyroid gland. Taurus Rising individuals are often described as physically sturdy, with a preference for steady rhythms in health and lifestyle. Some specific characteristics include:

Calm Demeanor: Taurus Rising tends to be patient, deliberate, and generally unhurried.

Affinity for Sensual Pleasures: They have a keen appreciation for comfort, good food, pleasant sounds, warm touches, and may cling to routines that offer security.

Stability and Endurance: Once set on a course, Taurus rarely changes direction abruptly. The "fixed earth" nature suggests a methodical, persistent approach to both health regimens and life goals.

Medical astrologers link Taurus with possiblevulnerabilities in the throat, glandular system, and metabolism (including weight management or thyroid issues).

The slower metabolism often attributed to Taurus Rising can be beneficial for steady energy but may also predispose them to conditions like hypothyroidism, weight gain, or fluid retention, especially if dietary habits are unbalanced.

The Mother's Gestational Experience and Taurus Rising

Building on Lynn Koiner's observational work, mothers of Taurus Rising children commonly describe a prenatal period focused on **acquiring comforts**, exploring **creative or cultural pursuits**, and providing a **"nest" of pleasant stability**:

Seeking Comfort and Security: Mothers often mention they felt the need to nest, accumulate resources, or create a cozy home environment during pregnancy. This might involve buying or rearranging furniture, planning future financial stability, or simply indulging in,

comforting routines. Their contentment and sense of physical ease can imprint onto the fetus, laying the groundwork for Taurus Rising's calm and steady disposition.

Creative and Musical Exposure: Koiner observed that Taurus Rising mothers might immerse themselves in music, art, or cultural activities during gestation. In classical astrology, Venus symbolizes art and beauty; in Taurus, this can translate into repeated exposure to harmonious sounds, artistic expressions, and tactile creativity. Fetal hearing develops significantly in the second and third trimesters, so the mother's preference for soothing music or art could shape the unborn child's sensory inclinations.

Emphasis on Physical Well-Being: Taurus Rising is all about the body, being comfortable in one's own skin. Mothers often monitor their diets carefully, ensuring that pregnancy is a period of **stable, healthy nourishment** for themselves and the fetus.

This pursuit of equilibrium and consistency may program the child to value bodily comfort and routine from day one.

Concerns with Resources: In many Taurus Rising stories, the parents are in the "acquisitional stage" of their relationship, building a home, saving money, or striving for financial security. These practical concerns might be internalized by the unborn child, creating an adult who seeks stability and can experience anxiety if financial or material security is threatened.

Modern Prenatal Research: Biological Underpinnings

From a scientific perspective, Taurus Rising's gestational narratives dovetail with findings that a stable, nurturing prenatal environment can shape a child's temperament and physiologic setpoints:

Maternal Calm and Cortisol Regulation:

When mothers experience relatively low stress during pregnancy, their cortisol levels tend to be more regulated.

This supports a calmer fetal environment, less stimulation of the fetal HPA (hypothalamic-pituitary-adrenal) axis.

Studies have shown that offspring exposed to consistently low to moderate maternal cortisol tend to develop stronger self-regulation skills, patience, and resilience. This aligns well with Taurus Rising's characteristic calm and stability.

Sensory Enrichment and Fetal Development:

Research indicates that fetal hearing becomes quite refined by the late second trimester, and a mother's preference for soothing music can reduce her stress levels, indirectly benefiting fetal development.

Some studies suggest that babies who experience rhythmic and melodic sounds in utero might show enhanced auditory processing and receptivity to music after birth. This parallels the creative, arts-appreciative nature frequently attributed to Taurus Rising (a sign ruled by Venus).

Nutritional Foundations and Metabolic Programming:

Modern science acknowledges "fetal programming" of metabolism: if a mother has a balanced diet and consistent nutrient intake, the fetus's metabolism learns "abundance" and stable rhythms, potentially reducing the risk of metabolic disorders later.

A calm, well-nourished prenatal environment might prime the child for slower, more deliberate growth patterns, which fits with Taurus's earth-bound, measured approach to life.

Maternal Positive Emotion and Fetal Well-Being:

When mothers focus on creating a comfortable, pleasant environment, surrounding themselves with beauty, emotional support, and stable finances, they experience lower anxiety and produce oxytocin, known as the "bonding hormone."

Oxytocin can cross the placenta in small amounts, promoting fetal calm. Over time, a fetus regularly exposed

to maternal oxytocin and low stress might emerge with a predisposition toward secure attachment and even "slower, more grounded" emotional patterns, reflections of a Taurus Rising temperament.

Taurus Rising in Adulthood: Health and Emotional Patterns

By adulthood, Taurus Rising individuals often embody the **patient, pleasure-oriented** approach established in the womb. Some key traits include:

Physical Grounding: A strong connection to the body can lead to mindful practices such as yoga, gardening, or savoring good meals. They tend to be aware of physical sensations and can excel in fields that require **practical know-how** or steady handling of resources.

Steadfast Emotional Nature: Taurus Rising folks usually maintain a calm, even-tempered demeanor. They prefer stability and may resist change, reflecting early prenatal experiences of **comfort and security**. They are also loyal and caring, though, when deeply provoked,

they can display a formidable stubborn streak.

Potential Metabolic Challenges: While many enjoy robust health, they should watch for thyroid imbalances, weight fluctuations, or issues with the throat and sinuses. They thrive on regular routines and can be sensitive to drastic dietary changes or chaotic lifestyles.

Sensitivity to Sensory Overload: On the flip side, if denied the comfort or "creature habits" they crave, Taurus Rising people might become anxious or withdrawn. Their strong Venusian desire for harmony means high-stress or overly fast-paced environments can leave them feeling overwhelmed or resentful.

Practical Guidance for Taurus Rising Natives and Caregivers

Honor the Senses:
Engage in relaxing sensory experiences such as gentle music, warm baths, aromatherapy, or tactile hobbies. This nurtures Taurus Rising's intrinsic need for comfort.

For children, playing soothing music or encouraging hands-on activities (e.g., sculpting clay, baking) can help them develop confidence and maintain emotional equilibrium.

Maintain Steady Routines:

A structured daily rhythm, regular mealtimes, sleep schedules, and consistent exercise, prevents metabolic and emotional imbalances.

Sudden changes can be disruptive to Taurus Rising's innate need for stability; advanced notice and gradual adaptation ease transitions.

Healthy Indulgence:

Taurus Rising folks may adore fine foods and pleasant surroundings but should guard against excess. Emphasize balanced, nourishing meals that fulfill their craving for quality without compromising health.

Integrative practices, like mindful eating, ensure that they enjoy life's pleasures without slipping into overindulgence

or stagnation.

Empowerment Through Security:

For some Taurus Rising individuals, financial or emotional security directly impacts their sense of well-being. Encouraging good money management or stable relationships can reinforce self-worth and peace of mind.

Recognizing the link between security and self-esteem is key: supportive partnerships and stable resources allow their natural creativity and reliability to flourish.

Balancing Stubbornness and Adaptability:

Encourage a gentle openness to new ideas and experiences. While their grounded nature is a gift, mild flexibility can prevent stagnation.

Therapy or coaching that highlights "change as growth" can help them adapt without sacrificing the comfort and predictability they cherish.

Conclusion

Taurus Rising provides a window into how maternal comfort-seeking and creative exposure during pregnancy might shape a child's eventual affinity for stability, beauty, and security. Astrologically, this sign's association with Venus resonates with themes of harmony and gentle perseverance. Modern scientific findings affirm that a low-stress, sensory-rich prenatal environment can yield a child who values calm, thrives on routine, and may have a heightened aesthetic or musical sensibility.

Adulthood for Taurus Rising often centers around fostering that secure base—both externally, through a stable home and finances, and internally, through a grounded self-identity. Recognizing these gestational roots can offer profound insights into health tendencies (like thyroid or weight issues) and personality traits (loyal, steady, occasionally stubborn). By understanding the convergence of **maternal experiences, developmental science, and Venusian symbolism,**

we see how the tranquil rhythms of pregnancy might echo in a Taurus Rising individual's lifelong pursuit of comfort, consistency, and creative expression.

Chapter 3

Gemini Rising: Embracing Movement and Mental Stimulation in the Womb

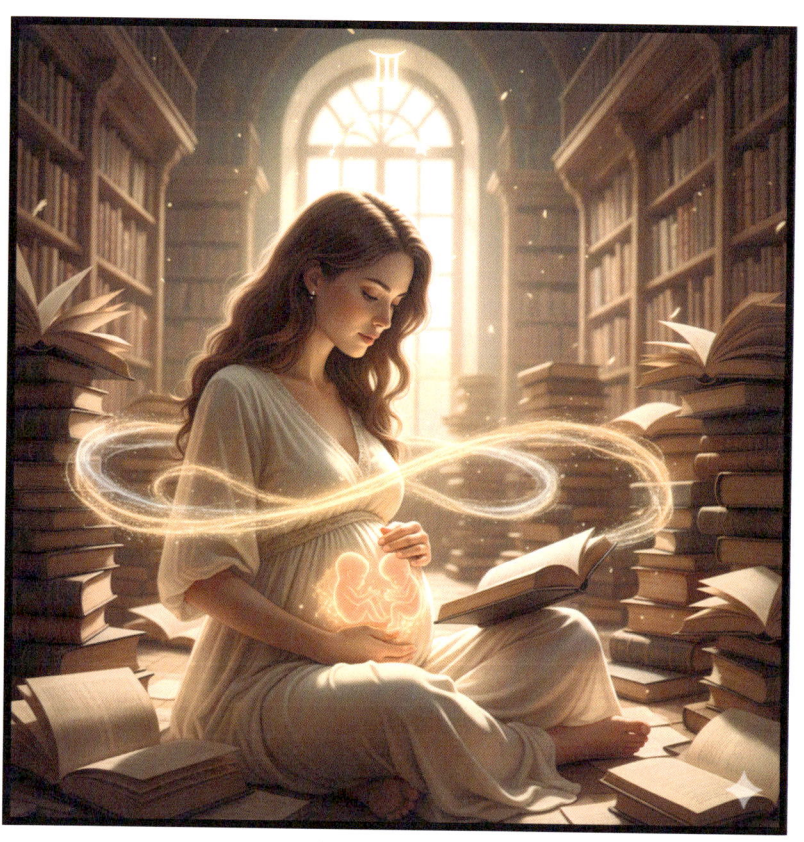

Introduction

Gemini is the third sign of the zodiac, ruled by Mercury, the planet of communication, curiosity, and swift change. Astrologically, those with Gemini Rising are typically described as adaptable, sociable, and eager to explore new ideas or environments. In the realm of medical astrology, Gemini correlates with the lungs, arms, hands, nervous system, and an overall affinity for movement and mental stimulation.

Just as Lynn Koiner's gestational theory proposes, the mother's experiences during pregnancy may lay the foundation for a child's future orientation, shaping the Ascendant's hallmark traits. For Gemini Rising, these prenatal impressions often revolve around movement, travel, changing scenery, and mental engagement. Modern scientific research on prenatal development suggests that a maternal environment filled with novelty, mobility, and intellectual stimulation can influence the fetus's neurological growth, potentially fostering flexibility and quickness in how the child will later learn and communicate.

29

Gemini Rising in Traditional Medical Astrology
Classical teachings link Gemini with:

The Respiratory System (lungs and bronchi):
Reflecting Mercury's connection to air, breath, and
communication.

Arms and Hands: Indicative of dexterity, manual skills,
and a restless urge to gesture or "do something."

The Nervous System: Reflecting mental agility and
adaptability, but also a potential predisposition to
nervous tension or overstimulation if not balanced.

From a medical standpoint, Gemini Rising individuals
can display a lively constitution, quick reflexes, and a
strong need for mental or physical novelty. However, they
may experience respiratory sensitivities (coughs,
bronchitis, sinus congestion), as well as stress-related
conditions linked to the nervous system (insomnia,
anxiety, or restlessness) if life becomes monotonous or
emotionally stifling.

The Mother's Gestational Experience and Gemini Rising According to Lynn Koiner's observations, mothers of Gemini Rising children often recall:

Frequent Movement or Travel: Some reported moving to a new home, traveling short distances regularly, or changing their daily routine multiple times while pregnant. Even something as simple as daily aerobics or consistent exercise can create a sense of restlessness and variety in the fetal environment.

Shifting Environments or Mental Stimulation: Gemini is governed by Mercury, a planet associated with learning and information exchange. Mothers might have pursued new subjects of study, read voraciously, or engaged in a fast-paced schedule. This intellectual "buzz" potentially imprints on the child in utero, laying the groundwork for Gemini Rising's trademark curiosity.

Adaptability Under Changing Circumstances: If the mother had to juggle multiple tasks, handle frequent errands, or coordinate changes in family routines,

the fetus may absorb an early lesson in flexibility. Gemini Rising children often arrive with an innate readiness to pivot and process fresh input, a skill that may trace back to their mother's varied experiences during pregnancy.

Social/Community Engagement: Some mothers reported increased social activity, visiting relatives, participating in local events, or hosting gatherings. The unborn child, immersed in a bustling social atmosphere, could later manifest the outgoing, talkative spirit often linked with Gemini Rising.

Modern Prenatal Research: Biological Underpinnings
While astrology uses symbolic language, modern science offers concrete mechanisms by which maternal mobility and mental stimulation may shape fetal development:

Neurological Stimulation and Learning:
The fetal brain is highly responsive to the mother's hormonal shifts triggered by stress, excitement, or cognitive engagement.

Moderate, positive stress (eustress) from varied activities can enhance neuroplasticity, leading to improved adaptability and information processing in the child.

Research suggests that babies born to mothers who engage in consistent learning or problem-solving activities during pregnancy may show stronger early cognitive markers, aligning with Gemini's mental agility.

Vestibular Stimulation from Movement:
The fetus perceives motion through the amniotic fluid and the mother's shifting center of gravity. Activities like regular exercise or traveling can stimulate the fetal vestibular system, potentially fostering a comfort with motion and change, an echo of Gemini's restless curiosity.

Some studies on prenatal movement and fetal well-being indicate that moderate maternal exercise helps regulate the fetal stress response, creating a child who is more resilient and adaptive to environmental shifts.

33

Respiratory Health and Maternal Breathing Patterns:

Gemini's link to the lungs is symbolically paralleled by the mother's respiratory rhythms. If a pregnant woman maintains healthy breathing practices (e.g., during aerobics or yoga), it can optimize fetal oxygenation.

Children whose mothers have healthy, steady respiratory patterns might be less prone to respiratory complications, although this is influenced by a host of other genetic and environmental factors.

Social Engagement and Language Exposure:

Several studies note that a fetus can hear muffled sounds by the third trimester, including the cadence and tone of the mother's voice. A mother who talks, reads aloud, or engages in lively conversation exposes the fetus to **early auditory patterns**.

This may lay groundwork for advanced language acquisition, reflecting the Mercury-ruled curiosity and communicativeness we associate with Gemini.

Gemini Rising in Adulthood: Health and Emotional Patterns

By adulthood, Gemini Rising often emerges as:

Adaptable and Mentally Active: Quick-witted and sociable, Gemini Rising individuals tend to thrive in fast-changing or intellectually stimulating environments. They may gravitate toward teaching, communications, journalism, or technology fields where variety is prized.

Restlessness and Potential for Overcommitment: If the formative environment taught them to handle multiple tasks, they can excel at multitasking but also risk mental overload or scattered energy. Balancing mental stimulation with moments of calm can prevent burnout.

Respiratory and Nervous System Watchpoints: They might be more vulnerable to **respiratory infections**, allergies, or seasonal issues like hay fever. On the nervous-system side, insomnia, anxiety, or tension headaches can flare up if they're mentally overstimulated or emotionally anxious.

Socially Connected Yet Detached: Gemini Rising thrives on information exchange and meeting people. However, if emotional depth or continuity is lacking, they can appear detached or superficial. Learning to sustain deeper emotional connections and moderate the "variety obsession" helps integrate their lively curiosity into stable relationships.

Practical Guidance for Gemini Rising Natives and Caregivers

Channel Curiosity in Healthy Ways:

Encourage diverse interests and hands-on learning, but introduce organization (like journaling or mind-mapping) to keep the mental sphere cohesive.

Gemini Rising children, for instance, benefit from interactive activities that let them absorb information while also teaching them to focus.

Support Balanced Routines:

Scheduled quiet or "unplugged" times can prevent mental hyperactivity.

Techniques such as breathwork, meditation, or restorative yoga help steady the nervous system.

Make room for spontaneity, Gemini thrives on novelty, but establish a core routine to avoid chronic stress or exhaustion.

Mindful Breathing and Respiratory Care:
Because Gemini is linked with the lungs, regular outdoor walks or gentle aerobic exercise can maintain respiratory health.

Individuals prone to respiratory allergies might explore preventative measures (e.g., air purifiers, herbal teas, or inhalation therapy).

Managing Information Overload:
Offer tools for digital detox or setting boundaries around social media/news intake, so that Mercury's mental energy doesn't become overwhelming.
Incorporate journaling, artistic expression, or discussion groups to convert swirling thoughts into coherent ideas.

Emphasize Communication Skills:

Gemini Rising people often need to talk things out, verbally process ideas, and engage in lively debates. Encourage healthy communication, whether it's through therapy, friendship circles, or intellectual clubs.

Conflicts can arise if they feel stifled or misunderstood. Teaching them to listen as well as speak fosters more meaningful exchanges.

Conclusion

Gemini Rising underscores how movement, mental stimulation, and shifting environments during pregnancy can imprint an energetic, curious, and adaptive nature on the developing child. In Lynn Koiner's prenatal theory, the mother's experiences of travel, exercise, study, or social bustle reflect key Mercury themes, mobility, flexibility, and communication, that become woven into the child's Ascendant.

From a medical-astrological vantage, Gemini Rising ,

corresponds to a strong mental acuity, a natural curiosity, and potential vulnerabilities in the respiratory and nervous systems.

Modern developmental researchsupports the idea that vestibular and cognitive stimulation in utero influences how a child's brain processes novelty, stress, and communication. By understanding these prenatal foundations, Gemini Rising individuals can harmonize their love of variety with a stable framework, reaping the benefits of a flexible mind while maintaining holistic well-being. Through practices like breathwork, structured routines, and deliberate downtime, they harness Gemini's swift mental energy to its fullest, living out their cosmic birthright of perpetual curiosity and vibrant exchange.

Chapter 4

Cancer Rising: Nurturing and Emotional Currents in the Womb

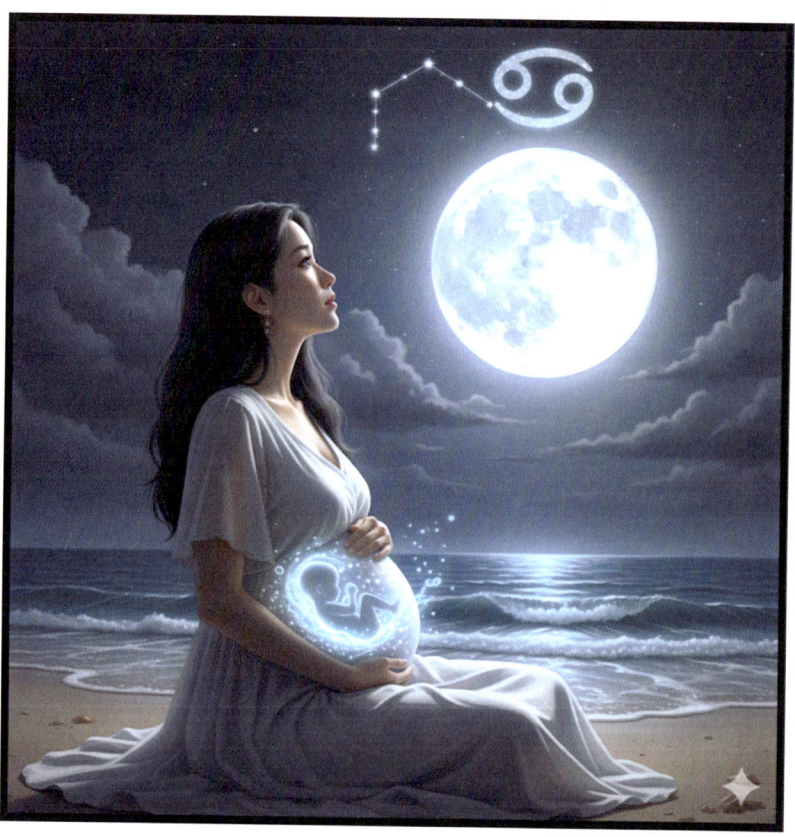

Introduction

Cancer, the fourth sign of the zodiac, is ruled by the Moon, a celestial body associated with maternal energy, emotional sensitivity, and instinctive nurturing. In astrology, Cancer Rising individuals typically display warmth, empathy, and a keen responsiveness to their immediate environment. However, they can also be prone to mood fluctuations and heightened sensitivity.

Following Lynn Koiner's prenatal theory, the mother's experiences and emotional climate during pregnancy profoundly shape Cancer Rising traits. When the mother undergoes pronounced emotional highs and lows, or experiences strong protective or nurturing instincts, the unborn child may internalize these patterns as the lens through which they engage with the outside world. Modern developmental science reinforces the idea that maternal emotional states, particularly stress, anxiety, or a sense of comfort, have a lasting impact on the fetus's physiological and emotional regulation. Cancer Rising, then, represents a compelling intersection of lunar symbolism and scientific evidence that early experiences,

in the womb help determine how we bond, feel, and adapt throughout life.

Cancer Rising in Traditional Medical Astrology
Classical teachings link Cancer with:

The Stomach, Breasts, and Digestive Processes: Cancer's emphasis on nourishment and security places the digestive system at center stage, both as a source of comfort and as a potential site of somatic stress (like "butterflies in the stomach").

The Fluid Body and Emotional States: Ruled by the Moon, Cancer is said to govern bodily fluids, including lymph and possibly hormonal fluctuations. Emotional tides can manifest physically in water retention or digestive disturbances.

Heightened Sensitivity and Receptivity: Cancer Rising people are often highly attuned to the emotional undercurrents in a room. This receptivity can be an asset but can also lead to overstimulation or anxiety if boundaries are not well-developed.

In medical astrology, these qualities mean that Cancer Rising individuals may need to pay special attention to digestion, fluid balance, and stress management to maintain physical and emotional well-being. They often feel their emotions "in their stomach" more directly than other signs, sometimes leading to issues like acid reflux, ulcers, or chronic indigestion when under strain.

The Mother's Gestational Experience and Cancer Rising
According to Lynn Koiner's research and observations:

Emotional Sensitivity or Moodiness: Many mothers of Cancer Rising children report experiencing significant emotional fluctuations during pregnancy. This might include **morning sickness, mood swings, or deep emotional sensitivity**, all of which the fetus may internalize, resulting in the child's heightened ability to pick up on subtle feelings.

Nurturing or Overprotective Concerns: Cancer symbolizes maternal protectiveness. Some mothers recall becoming extremely cautious about diet, environment, or

stressors while pregnant. This attitude of "I must take care of my baby at all costs" may instill in the unborn child a strong sense of security, or, if taken to an extreme, an anxious over-reliance on external nurturance.

Family and Domestic Focus: Because Cancer rules the home, the pregnancy period sometimes involves intense family involvement or domestic reorganization (e.g., renovating the nursery, moving closer to extended family, or seeking to create a cozy, protective nest). The baby then arrives "programmed" to value home and a sense of emotional belonging.

Stomach-Related Distress: Koiner notes that Cancer Rising mothers frequently mention significant morning sickness. The fetus is thus exposed to maternal digestive discomfort and emotional stress, which may translate into a child who later demonstrates stomach sensitivities and an acute attunement to emotional states.

Modern Prenatal Research: Biological Underpinnings Science underscores the ways maternal emotions and,

stressors while pregnant. This attitude of "I must take care of my baby at all costs" may instill in the unborn child a strong sense of security, or, if taken to an extreme, an anxious over-reliance on external nurturance.

Family and Domestic Focus: Because Cancer rules the home, the pregnancy period sometimes involves intense family involvement or domestic reorganization (e.g., renovating the nursery, moving closer to extended family, or seeking to create a cozy, protective nest). The baby then arrives "programmed" to value home and a sense of emotional belonging.

Stomach-Related Distress: Koiner notes that Cancer Rising mothers frequently mention significant morning sickness. The fetus is thus exposed to maternal digestive discomfort and emotional stress, which may translate into a child who later demonstrates stomach sensitivities and an acute attunement to emotional states.

Modern Prenatal Research: Biological Underpinnings
Science underscores the ways maternal emotions and,

45

Maternal Stress and Gut-Brain Axis:

High stress or emotional upheavals during pregnancy increase levels of cortisol and inflammatory markers, which can affect the fetal gut-brain axis. Emerging research links prenatal stress to gastrointestinal sensitivities in children, reflecting Cancer's digestive vulnerabilities.

Infants exposed to maternal stress hormones in utero can show a heightened stress reactivity postnatally, aligning with the Cancer Rising tendency toward emotional sensitivity.

Hormonal Environment and Emotional Regulation:

The Moon's symbolism around fluid regulation parallels scientific observations that changes in maternal estrogen, progesterone, and oxytocin can influence how the fetus's developing brain processes bonding and security.

If the mother experiences strong bursts of nurturant hormones (like oxytocin), the child may emerge with,

greater capacity for empathy and attachment, mirroring Cancer's caring nature.

Nausea and Gastrointestinal Imprinting:

Significant morning sickness or digestive issues can lead to shifts in **maternal-fetal nutrient flow**. While typically resolved by mid-pregnancy, these disruptions may teach the fetus (in a biochemical sense) about the volatility of bodily comfort.

This aligns with anecdotal reports of Cancer Rising children showing **sensitive stomachs**, food aversions, or emotional eating patterns.

Emotional Bonding and Attachment:

Studies on **prenatal attachment** suggest that mothers who actively bond with their babies in utero, talking to them, daydreaming about them, or simply holding them in a nurturing mental space, can foster stronger emotional security in the child. Cancer Rising is said to excel at emotional connection, suggesting this sign's link to strong prenatal bonding.

Cancer Rising in Adulthood: Health and Emotional Patterns

Once grown, Cancer Rising individuals often exhibit:

Deep Emotional Responsiveness: They can sense subtle shifts in others' moods, sometimes becoming the caretaker or "emotional sponge" of the group. This can be profoundly supportive but may also lead to empathic overload if they lack boundaries.

Protective and Home-Oriented: Their living space is a sanctuary. They may invest in comfy surroundings and prefer stable routines that provide emotional safety. If threatened, Cancer Rising can withdraw or become defensive, reflecting the crab's protective shell.

Digestive Sensitivities: Under stress, physical symptoms (stomach aches, bloating, changes in appetite) can flare up. Cancer Rising individuals do well when they address emotional tensions early, rather than allowing them to "sink into" the gut.

Mood Cycles Tied to External Events: Ruled by the Moon, Cancer Rising people might experience swings in energy and emotion that parallel lunar phases or changes in their environment. Recognizing these cycles can help them find rhythm and self-acceptance.

Strong Nurturing Instincts: They excel at creating emotional security for others, often in fields like caregiving, counseling, hospitality, or food services. Their predisposition for emotional labor can become a vocation or, if unchecked, a source of overextension.

Practical Guidance for Cancer Rising Natives and Caregivers
Nurture Emotional Boundaries:
Develop practices to **discharge absorbed emotions**, like journaling, mindfulness meditation, or creative expression (painting, music).

Recognize when you are taking on others' feelings too intensely. Setting compassionate limits can preserve well-being.

Gut-Friendly Lifestyle Choices:

Maintain a balanced diet that supports digestive health, whole grains, fermented foods, and adequate hydration. Emotional eating can be a pitfall; mindful eating routines help Cancer Rising differentiate between true hunger and stress-based cravings.

Stress-management techniques (yoga, breathwork, gentle exercise) can reduce digestive flare-ups.

Honor the Need for Security:

Seek or create comfortable home environments that provide emotional grounding. Simple choices like soft lighting, cozy furnishings, and personal mementos can enhance the sense of sanctuary.

When life demands change, proceed with gentle steps. Gradual transitions, rather than abrupt disruptions, align with Cancer Rising's preference for emotional safety.

Engage in Healthy Caregiving:

Cancer Rising often finds fulfillment in nurturing roles,

Family ties are usually significant. Fostering open communication and healthy boundaries with relatives helps maintain emotional balance.

Ride Emotional Waves Constructively:
Accept that shifting moods are part of the lunar temperament. Channel emotional energy into creative outlets, supportive relationships, or personal reflection time.

Embrace self-nurturing rituals, warm baths, gentle music, or evenings devoted to rest, just as one would care for a beloved child.

Conclusion
Cancer Rising arises from a prenatal environment deeply colored by **emotional currents, nurturing impulses, and sometimes digestive sensitivities**. These lunar themes often persist throughout the individual's life, manifesting as a profound empathy, a craving for emotional security, and a strong linkage between mood and physical well-being.

Family ties are usually significant. Fostering open communication and healthy boundaries with relatives helps maintain emotional balance.

Ride Emotional Waves Constructively:

Accept that shifting moods are part of the lunar temperament. Channel emotional energy into creative outlets, supportive relationships, or personal reflection time.

Embrace self-nurturing rituals, warm baths, gentle music, or evenings devoted to rest, just as one would care for a beloved child.

Conclusion

Cancer Rising arises from a prenatal environment deeply colored by **emotional currents, nurturing impulses, and sometimes digestive sensitivities**. These lunar themes often persist throughout the individual's life, manifesting as a profound empathy,

a craving for emotional security, and a strong linkage between mood and physical well-being.

Contemporary findings on prenatal stress, hormone regulation, and maternal bonding mesh with Cancer's archetypal focus on care and comfort, reinforcing Lynn Koiner's notion that the Ascendant is partly shaped by how the mother experiences pregnancy. For Cancer Rising individuals, this can mean a highly attuned emotional life rooted in early exposure to maternal protectiveness or volatility. By understanding their predisposition toward empathy and digestion-linked mood responses, Cancer Rising natives can harness their capacity for deep connection in ways that nurture both themselves and others, honoring the imprint left on them from the very start of life.

Chapter 5

Leo Rising: Radiant Warmth and Self-Expression from the Womb

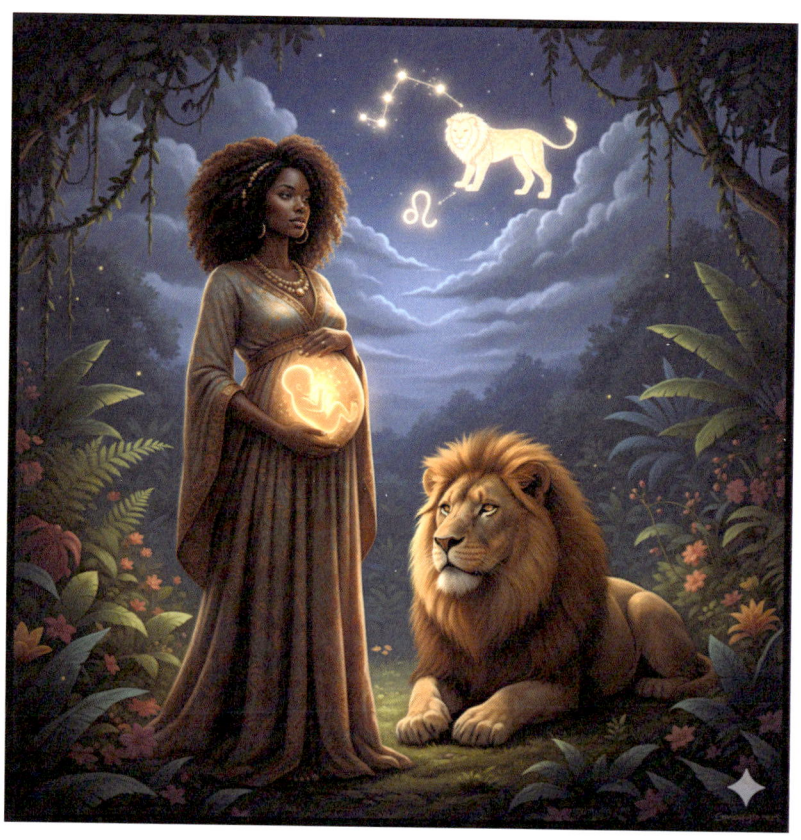

Introduction

Leo is the fifth sign of the zodiac, classically ruled by the Sun, a symbol of vitality, willpower, and creative self-expression. When placed on the Ascendant, Leo bestows a natural charisma and a flair for the dramatic, individuals with Leo Rising often exhibit confidence, warmth, and a strong desire to "stand out." Yet, as with all Rising Signs, medical astrologer Lynn Koiner contends that Leo's trademark boldness can begin in utero, shaped by the mother's pregnancy experiences.

In Koiner's research, mothers of Leo Rising children frequently reported receiving **a great deal of attention or praise while pregnant**, and this supportive, celebratory environment is believed to imprint the developing fetus with a sense of importance and stage presence. Modern developmental science, similarly, suggests that a mother's positive emotional state, social involvement, and thriving physical health can enhance fetal well-being, potentially leading to children who are more outgoing and self-assured.

In this chapter, we'll explore how these themes weave together, creating the distinctive aura of Leo Rising.

Leo Rising in Traditional Medical Astrology
From the standpoint of classical astrology, Leo Rising is linked to:

Heart and Circulatory System: Traditionally, Leo rules the heart, spine, and upper back. People with Leo Rising may have strong constitutions but should remain mindful of cardiovascular health, blood pressure, and stress management, particularly when they put themselves "out there" energetically.

Vitality and Warmth: Solar rulership highlights energy, generosity, and leadership qualities. Physically, Leo Rising individuals often manifest a commanding presence or notable posture. They can be physically robust but may experience **burnout** if they consistentlyoperate at full tilt.

Pride and Dignity: Leo energy emphasizes self-worth.

When balanced, it fuels healthy confidence; when unbalanced, it can lean toward vanity or obstinacy. This dynamic can extend into healthcare habits, as Leo Rising folks often take pride in physical appearance or performance but may resist advice they perceive as undermining their autonomy.

In medical astrology, the **Sun's** influence can also point to conditions involving **inflammation, fever**, or "overheating" if the individual runs themselves ragged. Overall, a strong will to shine or lead is often apparent early in life.

The Mother's Gestational Experience and Leo Rising
Lynn Koiner's observations highlight several common themes for mothers of Leo Rising children:

Receiving Positive Attention: The mother may have been complimented frequently on her appearance or "pregnancy glow," reinforcing a sense of prestige. Family, friends, and even strangers might have gone out of their way to express admiration or provide assistance.

This environment of enthusiastic support can cultivate an in-womb template of **"I am special"** for the unborn child.

Experiencing Enhanced Self-Confidence: Many mothers recall feeling unusually good about themselves during pregnancy, sometimes describing it as a period of robust health and personal empowerment. This heightened self-esteem could be internalized by the fetus as an **optimistic blueprint**, later emerging as the Leo Rising inclination to shine confidently in social settings.

Increased Social Engagement: Because Leo is a socially expressive sign, the mother might have attended more social gatherings or garnered special attention in her community, an environment that fosters the unborn child's sense of participation and recognition. The pregnancy itself can become a "spotlight" experience, mirroring Leo's stage-loving nature.

Potential Outer Planet Overlays: During certain years, planets like Pluto or Transpluto were transiting ,

Leo. If these made a strong contact with the Ascendant, they could modify the classic "regal" patterns, introducing themes of **power struggles, self-sufficiency, or perfectionism**. Even so, the core sense of solar importance remains prominent.

Modern Prenatal Research: Biological Underpinnings

Contemporary scientific studies support the idea that **positive maternal mood, social connection, and physical vitality** can have profound effects on fetal development:

Maternal Well-Being and Dopamine Pathways:

A pregnant mother's sense of joy or self-confidence can raise levels of **dopamine and endorphins**, improving her overall mood and stress resilience.

These positive biochemical states may "communicate" to the fetus that the world is safe and abundant, encouraging a predisposition toward **outgoing social behavior**, an analog to Leo Rising's sunny disposition.

Social Support as a Buffer:

High levels of social support, friends checking in, family giving compliments or practical help, have been shown to lower maternal cortisol, a stress hormone. Babies born to mothers with strong social networks often exhibit higher self-regulation and sociability.

Leo Rising's characteristic need for recognition and affirmation might reflect an intrauterine memory of maternal emotional buoyancy and social connectedness.

Positive Emotions and Cardiovascular Health:

If the mother stays active and maintains good cardiovascular health, it can translate to healthier fetal heart development. This resonates with Leo's traditional rulership of the heart and circulation.

Feeling physically vibrant may also reduce pregnancy complications, setting the stage for a baby who inherits robust vitality.

Identity and Self-Expression:

Some research indicates that mothers who experience heightened self-awareness and empowerment during pregnancy often communicate more with the fetus, singing, speaking, or daydreaming about future aspirations.

Such prenatal "dialogue" can foster an early sense of identity formation in the child. In astrological terms, the "solar seeds" planted might grow into that Leo Rising flair for self-expression.

Leo Rising in Adulthood: Health and Emotional Patterns
As adults, Leo Rising individuals often embody:

Charismatic Presence: They're quick to take leadership roles, comfortable in the limelight, and frequently serve as the "heart" of social situations. They thrive in environments where they can entertain, organize, or inspire.

Vulnerability to Overextension: The desire to maintain an image of strength and confidence can lead to,

burnout. Leo Rising may push themselves beyond healthy limits, particularly if they feel that stepping back would diminish their "star quality."

Heart and Spine Watchpoints: True to the sign's domain, paying attention to cardiovascular health, posture, and back care is important. Stress management techniques that calm the entire system (e.g., moderate exercise, yoga, or mindful relaxation) help offset risks associated with over-activation.

The Need for Acknowledgment: Affirmation is like fuel for Leo Rising. They flourish when their contributions are noticed and praised. Without recognition, they can fall into self-doubt or pride-driven conflict.

Generosity and Protective Instincts: Leo Rising individuals can be tremendously warm and loyal, often taking younger peers or loved ones under their wing. When channeled positively, their leadership qualities can uplift others rather than overshadow them.

Practical Guidance for Leo Rising Natives and Caregivers

Moderate the Spotlight:

Encourage healthy self-expression, performing arts, leadership clubs, or volunteer efforts, but balance it with downtime. Teaching them that stepping out of the limelight at times isn't a loss of status can prevent exhaustion.

Engage in creative hobbies (painting, singing, drama) that let them shine while providing a structured outlet for their expansive energy.

Foster Heart Health Early:

For children, ample **outdoor play** and age-appropriate sports build strong cardiovascular foundations. As they grow, mindful exercise routines help maintain a robust circulatory system.

Encourage a **balanced diet** and awareness of stress triggers to prevent the buildup of tension that can impact the heart or spine.

Affirmation and Emotional Validation:

Leo Rising thrives on positive feedback. Offer sincere praise for genuine achievements to build healthy self-esteem.

Balanced feedback is key: let them know you admire their passion, but also encourage humility, teamwork, and empathy for others.

Self-Awareness Around Ego and Pride:

Teach children (and adults) how to handle criticism gracefully. Modeling that self-worth does not depend solely on external applause fosters emotional resilience.

In therapy or personal development work, focusing on unconditional self-love can help them channel Leo's warmth and leadership without tipping into arrogance.

Connection to Inner Child:

Leo Rising often has a playful streak. Maintaining a sense of **fun, creativity, and spontaneity** into adulthood keeps them vibrant.

64

Give them space to explore theater, dance, or public speaking in safe, supportive environments, this nurtures the cosmic "star" within.

Conclusion

Leo Rising emerges from a gestational setting defined by **admiration, warmth, and a sense of personal significance**. Mothers who felt vibrant, socially supported, and praised during pregnancy passed along an aura of positivity that the Leo Rising child later weaves into their persona. Traditional medical astrology aligns this sign with solar energy, the heart, and a powerful drive to lead, while modern prenatal research corroborates the benefits of strong social networks, maternal well-being, and enhanced fetal development.

By recognizing these origins, Leo Rising individuals can cultivate health through **balanced self-expression, stress management, and genuine self-love**.

They enter the world with an innate desire to shine, and, when guided by humility and empathy, they can light up the lives of others with a generous, radiant glow.

Chapter 6

Virgo Rising: Precision, Well-Being, and the Gestational Call to Service

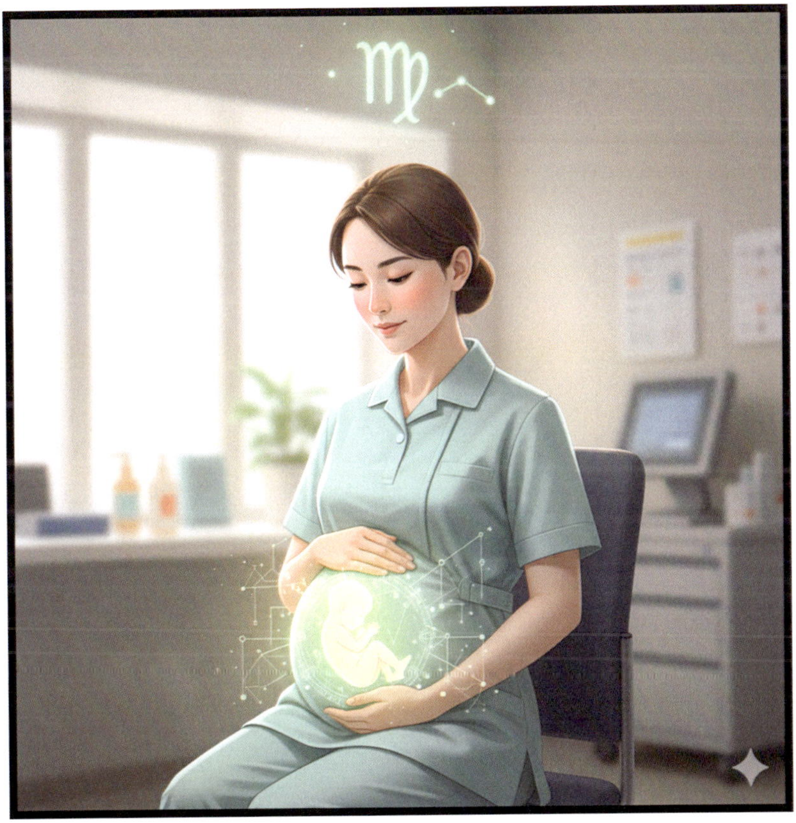

Introduction

Virgo is the sixth sign of the zodiac, classically ruled by Mercury, which governs communication, analysis, and detail orientation. When Virgo appears on the Ascendant, individuals often develop a keen eye for organization, healthful routines, and practical service to others. According to medical astrologer Lynn Koiner's prenatal theory, this meticulous, service-driven temperament can be shaped by the mother's experience of pregnancy, particularly if she was more guarded about her health, fixated on details, or diligent in her self-care.

From a medical astrology vantage point, Virgo Rising is associated with the digestive system, the assimilation of nutrients, and a careful approach to bodily well-being. Contemporary research supports the notion that the mother's careful attention to diet, prenatal check-ups, and general routines can imprint the fetus with a predisposition toward diligence, conscientiousness, and health awareness. This chapter delves into how that gestational environment might give rise to Virgo Rising's characteristic analytical mindset.

Virgo Rising in Traditional Medical Astrology

Virgo has been linked to:

The Digestive and Intestinal Tract: Virgo Rising individuals may be especially attuned to dietary factors, gut health, and issues like food sensitivities or irritable bowel syndrome (IBS).

A Focus on Health and Hygiene: Virgo is often depicted as the sign of purity and order. When on the Ascendant, it contributes to a methodical approach to nutrition, cleanliness, and daily habits.

Analytical Skills and Attention to Detail: With Mercury as the planetary ruler, Virgo Rising tends to process information thoroughly, sometimes resulting in perfectionistic tendencies.

Health-wise, Virgo Ascendants can be both physically resilient (due to careful habits) and vulnerable to psychosomatic complaints, especially if anxiety or an overactive "critical mind" generates stress in the body. Finding balance between **self-improvement** and **self-**

acceptance is a central theme for Virgo Rising.

The Mother's Gestational Experience and Virgo Rising
Based on Lynn Koiner's observations:

Attention to Health and Diet: Many mothers of Virgo Rising children recall **meticulous self-care** during pregnancy, watching their diet, sticking to strict supplement regimens, or engaging in consistent exercise. Their caution and desire to avoid complications can pass a sense of "the importance of details" to the developing fetus.

Heightened Worry or Fussiness: Some mothers describe feeling anxious about "doing everything right," especially if they'd had previous miscarriages or complications. This ingrained cautiousness, sometimes bordering on worry, may later manifest in the child as a **hyper-vigilant** or **perfectionistic** streak.

Routine and Consistency: The mother might have been very routine-oriented, keeping the same meal times,

bedtimes, or prenatal appointments with clockwork precision. Such a steady environment can program the unborn child for predictability, aligning with Virgo Rising's comfort in structured routines.

Practical Problem-Solving: Virgo is a service-oriented sign. Mothers often report tackling small details, like organizing the nursery with extra care or fixing every minor household glitch, throughout the pregnancy. The child may enter life "knowing" that detail-oriented service is a natural expression of care and love.

Modern Prenatal Research: Biological Underpinnings
Scientific findings offer plausible mechanisms for how a mother's thoroughness and possible anxiety might shape fetal development:

Maternal Stress and the Gut-Brain Axis:
If the mother is **chronically worried** about potential risks, her cortisol levels might be elevated. However, in modest amounts, concern can also motivate **positive,**

health-promoting behaviors (like proper nutrition and medical checkups).

Research indicates that maternal worry can influence **fetal stress reactivity**, potentially leading to a child predisposed to careful (sometimes anxious) vigilance.

Nutritional Programming:

Virgo's emphasis on diet aligns with scientific evidence that **consistent prenatal nutrition** supports the fetus's digestive system and metabolism. Babies born under these circumstances often display **steady growth patterns** and may show fewer nutritional deficiencies early in life.

The child may develop a natural inclination toward **healthful eating** or an interest in food quality and purity, paralleling Virgo's desire for cleanliness and order.

Habit Formation and Neural Pathways:

The mother's adherence to **regular schedules** could,

health-promoting behaviors (like proper nutrition and medical checkups).

Research indicates that maternal worry can influence **fetal stress reactivity**, potentially leading to a child predisposed to careful (sometimes anxious) vigilance.

Nutritional Programming:

Virgo's emphasis on diet aligns with scientific evidence that **consistent prenatal nutrition** supports the fetus's digestive system and metabolism. Babies born under these circumstances often display **steady growth patterns** and may show fewer nutritional deficiencies early in life.

The child may develop a natural inclination toward **healthful eating** or an interest in food quality and purity, paralleling Virgo's desire for cleanliness and order.

Habit Formation and Neural Pathways:

The mother's adherence to **regular schedules** could ,

73

contribute to more predictable hormonal rhythms (including melatonin and cortisol), which the fetus experiences as well.

Some studies suggest that children who experience in utero consistency may exhibit better self-regulation and adaptability to routines post-birth, mirroring Virgo Rising's methodical nature.

Cognitive Influences:

Pregnant mothers who remain mentally active, detail-focused, or engaged in "left-brain" tasks (planning, organizing, studying) may modulate their own **dopamine and norepinephrine levels**, indirectly shaping fetal neurological development.

This environment might prime the child for **analytical thinking** and a strong orientation to problem-solving, aligning closely with Virgo's Mercury rulership.

Virgo Rising in Adulthood: Health and Emotional Patterns

By adulthood, Virgo Rising individuals often display:

Refined Routine and Lifestyle: They prefer an orderly schedule and can be disciplined with exercise, diet, or daily tasks. Small deviations may cause them undue stress if they're not careful to cultivate flexibility.

Critical Mindset, Positives and Pitfalls: Their analytical skill can excel in careers that demand precision (e.g., research, healthcare, systems management). However, they risk slipping into self-criticism or over-analysis, leading to anxiety or procrastination.

Digestive Sensitivities: A direct outcome of their prenatal "health imprint" may be a highly responsive gut, correlating with psychosomatic issues (e.g., upset stomach during emotional distress). Maintaining balanced, mindful eating is crucial.

Service Orientation: Virgo Rising adults often find fulfillment in helping, fixing, or organizing for the sake of others.

While this is admirable, it can become a burden if they fail to set boundaries or practice self-care.

Strong Work Ethic: They take pride in doing tasks thoroughly, sometimes setting the bar extremely high. When recognized, this diligence brings them deep satisfaction, aligning with their internal drive for mastery and usefulness.

Practical Guidance for Virgo Rising Natives and Caregivers

Balance Structure with Flexibility:
Embrace schedules but practice **"planned spontaneity"**, build in occasional free blocks of time to quell stress related to sudden changes.

Use organizational tools (lists, planners) while remaining open to unexpected shifts in routine.

Gut Health and Stress Management:

76

Prioritize nutritious, balanced meals and consider probiotics or dietary support if digestion is an ongoing issue.

Integrative methods such as **yoga, breathwork, or mindfulness** can help calm the nervous system and reduce stress manifestations in the gut.

Embrace Imperfection:
Teach children (and remind adults) that mistakes are part of growth. Small "flaws" in a project or meal do not negate the effort.

Journaling or therapy can gently reframe perfectionistic tendencies, encouraging self-compassion.

Harness Analytical Strengths:
Virgo Rising excels at research, detail work, and systems organization, nurture these gifts in healthy ways (clubs, study groups, or skill-building workshops).

Encourage them to delegate tasks at times, ensuring they,

do not shoulder every detail alone.

Meaningful Service:

Many Virgo Rising individuals thrive in helping roles, medical, educational, environmental, or humanitarian. Finding a purposeful channel for this service impetus prevents bottled-up frustration.

Remind them that self-care is as essential as caring for others.

Conclusion

Virgo Rising represents the synergy between meticulous prenatal experiences and an adult life guided by discernment, service, and health consciousness. Mothers who conscientiously monitored their own well-being during pregnancy, perhaps after prior complications or simply out of a desire for perfection, could impart these exacting standards to the developing fetus. Modern science parallels this dynamic, showing how measured maternal worry, diligent self-care, and consistent routines

can "program" a child for conscientious behavior and a deep interest in holistic well-being.

With Virgo on the Ascendant, individuals grow into diligent caregivers, both to themselves and to others, though they must learn to temper perfectionism and address psychosomatic vulnerabilities. By embracing their carefully cultivated instincts while practicing flexibility, self-compassion, and balanced living, Virgo Rising natives can use their analytic gifts and service mindset to contribute profoundly to their communities and personal relationships.

Chapter 7

Libra Rising: Seeking Harmony and Balance from the Womb

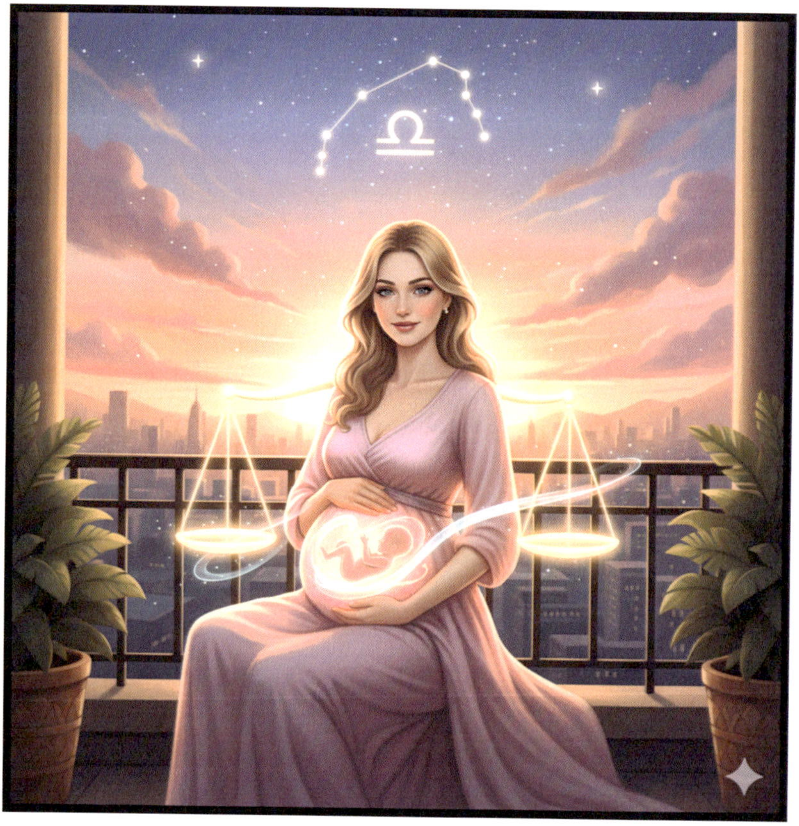

Introduction

Libra, the seventh sign of the zodiac, is Venus-ruled and renowned for themes of balance, beauty, and cooperation. With Libra on the Ascendant, individuals often develop social grace, a keen aesthetic sense, and a powerful drive to maintain equilibrium in their relationships. According to medical astrologer Lynn Koiner's prenatal theory, this emphasis on balance can be traced back to the mother's experiences during pregnancy, especially if she strove to harmonize competing needs, preserve peaceful environments, or show heightened concern for fair treatment.

From a medical astrology perspective, Libra Rising is associated with the kidneys (organs that maintain the body's fluid balance) and the body's overall equilibrium. Modern scientific research on prenatal development further supports the idea that maternal stress regulation, social relationships, and emotional well-being can shape a child's tendency toward diplomacy, fairness, or conflict-avoidance.

Libra Rising in Traditional Medical Astrology
Libra is classically connected with:

Kidneys and Lower Back: Libra Rising individuals may be susceptible to kidney-related issues (e.g., imbalances in fluid processing, kidney infections) and lower-back discomfort, particularly during times of stress.

Endocrine System and Hormonal Equilibrium: A balanced internal environment is part of Libra's core symbolism; disruptions to hormonal harmony can affect mood stability and physical well-being.

Aesthetics and Diplomacy: Ruled by Venus, Libra imbues a refined appreciation for art, beauty, and harmonious social interaction. Physically, Libra Rising individuals often have a graceful demeanor and a desire for calm, elegant surroundings.

Though typically well-poised, Libra Rising can become anxious or indecisive when faced with conflict or imbalance.

Striving to maintain outer peace, they may downplay their own needs, sometimes causing hidden stress that can manifest in physical tension or kidney/adrenal strain.

The Mother's Gestational Experience and Libra Rising
Based on Lynn Koiner's observations:

Emphasis on Harmony: Mothers often reported going to great lengths to keep life in balance during pregnancy. This might include smoothing over conflicts, decorating or reorganizing spaces to create beauty, or dedicating extra time to creative outlets like music or floral arrangements.

Conflict-Avoidance and People-Pleasing: Some mothers suppressed personal frustrations for the sake of household peace, potentially instilling the unborn child with a subconscious habit of avoiding confrontation or sacrificing personal needs to keep others happy.

Balanced Emotional Tone: If the mother succeeded in preserving harmony, the fetus may receive consistent,

signals of tranquility, leading to a child predisposed to calm, diplomatic behavior. However, if the mother's harmonious façade masked unresolved tension, the child might sense the underlying stress, emerging with heightened anxiety around discord.

Artistic or Social Engagement: Koiner notes that Libra Rising is often accompanied by strong artistic or social influences during gestation, listening to lovely music, attending cultural events, or seeking out aesthetically pleasing environments. The fetus thus "learns" to associate beauty and social grace with safety.

Modern Prenatal Research: Biological Underpinnings
Contemporary science suggests that maternal **emotional balance, social support, and stress regulation** all significantly influence fetal development:

Stress and the HPA Axis:
When a mother strives for serenity, she may keep cortisol levels more stable, buffering the fetus from extreme stress-hormone fluctuations.

This fosters moderate stress reactivity in the child, aligning with Libra's preference for calm and collaboration.

However, if the mother represses conflict while still experiencing internal turmoil, the fetus can still sense elevated stress markers, potentially leading the child to heightened sensitivity toward interpersonal tension.

Emotional Regulation and Conflict Management:
Research on **maternal-fetal emotional regulation** indicates that a mother who navigates stress calmly (or channels it productively, e.g., through creative pursuits) passes on more adaptive coping strategies to her child.

Libra Rising's diplomatic style may partly reflect these in-womb lessons in **conflict de-escalation** and the pursuit of external peace.

Social Bonds and Oxytocin:
Socially connected pregnant mothers, those who maintain supportive friendships or attend social events, may

produce more oxytocin, enhancing trust and bonding. Babies born to these mothers might be more socially attuned, paralleling Libra's interpersonal focus.

If the mother focuses on art, beauty, and emotional well-being, she may maintain an elevated "feel-good" hormonal state, encouraging the fetus to associate calm, gracious behavior with safety.

Kidney and Fluid Balance:
Libra's association with the kidneys resonates with research linking maternal hydration, electrolyte balance, and renal health to fetal development. Chronic dehydration or poor kidney function can increase pregnancy risks, indirectly affecting the fetus's baseline stress.

A mother who diligently monitors fluid intake and health might reduce strain on her own kidneys, thereby maintaining a more stable internal environment, potentially priming the child for the balanced "Libra vibe."

Libra Rising in Adulthood: Health and Emotional Patterns

By adulthood, Libra Rising individuals typically exhibit:

Diplomatic Social Skills: They are often skilled at reading group dynamics, facilitating compromise, and putting others at ease. This can be a strength in careers requiring negotiation, design, or public relations.

Desire for External Harmony: Libra Rising folks feel uncomfortable amid conflict. They may prioritize pleasing others or smoothing over disagreements to preserve harmony, even if doing so conflicts with their personal feelings.

Potential Indecisiveness: Their cardinal air quality (always seeking the "best option") can lead to **overthinking**. Fear of causing imbalance can render them hesitant about making firm choices.

Kidney/Adrenal Watchpoints: Physical stress can sometimes accumulate in the **lower back or kidney ,**

region. Good hydration, balanced diets, and timely relaxation help maintain equilibrium.

Aesthetics and Grace: Many Libra Rising adults have an innate sense of style or design. Whether through fashion, interior decorating, or fine arts, they channel their Venus-ruled love of beauty.

Practical Guidance for Libra Rising Natives and Caregivers

Healthy Conflict Resolution:
Encourage them to speak up about personal needs and emotions rather than burying them. Active listening and respectful debate help them gain confidence in addressing friction.

Remind them that genuine harmony involves both authentic expression and compromise, not one-sided sacrifice.

Fostering Decision-Making Skills:

Overthinking can delay important choices. Libra Rising benefits from structured decision-making, such as listing pros and cons, or setting time limits on deliberation.

Teaching children to trust their instincts while weighing facts can reduce stress and indecisiveness in later life.

Embrace Both Self and Social Balance:
While diplomacy is admirable, self-care must not be neglected. Set boundaries in relationships to avoid exhaustion from constant people-pleasing.

Mindful practices (e.g., yoga, tai chi) stabilize the mind-body equilibrium, supporting Libra's longing for internal and external harmony.

Kidney and Lower-Back Care:
Adequate hydration and a diet that supports electrolyte balance are crucial. Foods rich in potassium and magnesium may help maintain healthy kidney function.

Incorporate gentle stretching or core exercises to prevent,

lower-back strain. Massage or chiropractic care can relieve tension that builds up in this area.

Creative Outlets and Beautiful Environments:

Libra Rising individuals are nourished by art, music, and visually appealing surroundings. Encourage them to curate harmonious spaces (home, work) that soothe the senses.

Engaging with the arts, whether participating or simply appreciating, can be a potent form of stress relief and self-discovery.

Conclusion

Libra Rising emerges from a **gestational backdrop of harmony-seeking, emotional poise, and an emphasis on pleasing aesthetics**. Mothers who consciously or unconsciously avoided conflict and prioritized beauty or tranquility during pregnancy often imprint upon the fetus an affinity for balanced, diplomatic engagement with the world.

From a medical astrology viewpoint, Libra Rising is closely tied to the kidneys and bodily equilibrium, reflecting the sign's innate drive for internal and external harmony. Modern prenatal studies further validate how maternal emotional regulation, social support, and stable physiology can cultivate children who prefer cooperation and grace. As adults, Libra Rising natives excel at creating harmony but must remember that true balance includes advocating for themselves, not merely yielding to others. Through careful attention to conflict resolution, self-care, and artistic expression, they can uphold their signature poise while forging authentic connections in an ever-shifting social landscape.

Chapter 8

Scorpio Rising: Intensity, Transformation, and the Womb's Deep Emotions

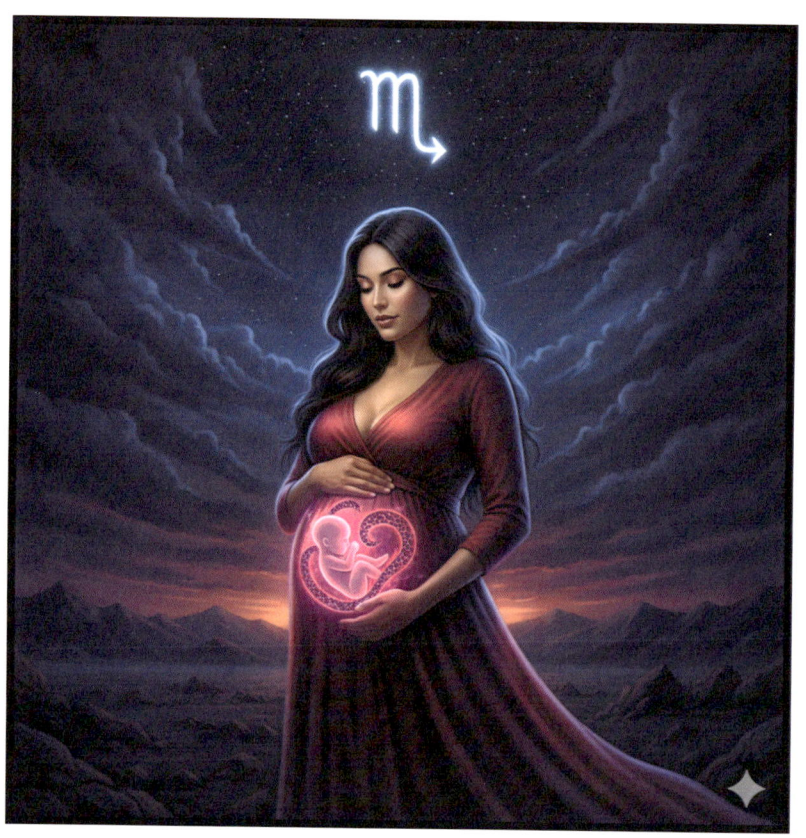

Introduction

Scorpio is the eighth sign of the zodiac, traditionally ruled by Mars (and, in modern astrology, co-ruled by Pluto). It symbolizes depth, intensity, and transformative power. When Scorpio appears on the Ascendant, individuals often project a magnetic aura, coupled with emotional perceptiveness and a desire for control or mastery over their environment. According to medical astrologer Lynn Koiner's prenatal theory, this powerful Scorpio energy can originate in the mother's experiences during pregnancy, especially if they involve profound emotional undercurrents, a sense of being out of control, or strong currents of resentment or secrecy.

Medical astrology assigns Scorpio rulership over the reproductive system, excretory system, and transformative processes in the body. Modern prenatal research supports the idea that maternal stress, secrecy, or tension during gestation can shape a child's heightened stress responses and a tendency toward deep emotional intensity.

In this chapter, we'll explore how these themes align, painting a picture of Scorpio Rising's psychological and physiological foundations.

Scorpio Rising in Traditional Medical Astrology
Classically, Scorpio is linked to:

The Reproductive Organs and Eliminative Systems: Scorpio Rising individuals may show sensitivity in the sexual organs, colon, bladder, and related areas. They often benefit from paying close attention to reproductive health and detoxification.

Issues of Control, Power, and Purging: Scorpio's transformative energy often involves probing beneath the surface. Scorpio Rising folks may experience intense emotional cycles, forging resilience but also prone to moments of power struggle.

Focus and Regeneration: When channeled positively, Scorpio Rising has a remarkable capacity for healing, renewal, and psychological insight. Physically, they can exhibit strong recuperative powers after illness.

Because Scorpio is a fixed water sign, the emotional depths of Scorpio Rising can be quite still on the surface but extremely intense underneath. This fixed quality lends persistence and an unyielding will once they commit to a path, whether for healing, ambition, or personal transformation.

The Mother's Gestational Experience and Scorpio Rising Drawing on Lynn Koiner's research and anecdotal evidence:

Heightened Emotional Turbulence: Scorpio or Pluto rising often indicates that the mother felt deep anger, resentment, fear, or stress during pregnancy. She may have resented the loss of control over her body, the constraints of family or finances, or an unwelcome intrusion by extended relatives. These tumultuous feelings can imprint an intense emotional backdrop on the unborn child.

Secrets or Suppressed Emotions: Sometimes, the pregnancy itself was kept secret or aspects of the situation

were hidden from others. The mother's desire to maintain privacy or conceal certain facts may correlate with the child's later tendency toward privacy, guardedness, or secrecy.

Overwhelming Desire to Retain Control: Many mothers described frustration at being "forced" into decisions or circumstances, mirroring Scorpio's aversion to feeling powerless. This can engender an unborn child who instinctively grapples with control issues or a fear of vulnerability.

Powerful Shifts and Transformations: On the flip side, some mothers found the pregnancy profoundly transformative, an emotional "rebirth" that helped them confront personal fears. Thus, the fetus might absorb not just anger or resentment but also the **alchemical process of change**, leading to Scorpio Rising's fierce resilience.

Modern Prenatal Research: Biological Underpinnings

Contemporary science provides clues for how maternal stress, secrecy, or strong emotional undercurrents might shape the fetus:

Chronic Stress and Cortisol Overexposure:

High, sustained levels of cortisol or adrenaline during pregnancy can re-tune a child's stress-response systems, potentially leading to heightened vigilance and intensity in emotional reactions. This resonates with Scorpio Rising's potent emotional landscape.

If the mother feels powerless or resentful, the fetus experiences biochemical markers of that negativity, possibly emerging with a **sensitive "fear/threat" radar**.

Emotional Repression and Epigenetic Imprints:

Research on epigenetics suggests that suppressed maternal emotions, especially trauma or ongoing tension, may modify gene expression in the fetus, influencing **stress adaptation** and emotional regulation.

This biological mechanism could explain Scorpio Rising's predisposition toward deeply buried feelings and transformational coping strategies.

Protective or Fear-Based Decision-Making:

Mothers who experience fear of external judgment or who face unsupportive environments might "armor up" psychologically. This can translate to a fetus that's primed to detect threats or sense the need for self-protection, key Scorpio themes.

Babies whose mothers felt compelled to keep personal matters hidden may develop enhanced emotional acuity, reading subtle cues of safety or danger in their environment.

Hormonal Tides of Transformation:

Pregnancy is inherently transformative; if the mother channels that energy into empowerment and deep healing, the fetus can benefit from a more purposeful and courageous imprint.

Some evidence suggests that mothers who confront and process their stress, rather than suppressing it, can moderate the potential adverse effects on fetal development, mirroring Scorpio's potential for regeneration after a crisis.

Scorpio Rising in Adulthood: Health and Emotional Patterns
Once grown, Scorpio Rising individuals often embody:

Deep Emotional Reservoirs: They might appear composed or mysterious externally, but they experience feelings, love, anger, passion, with heightened intensity. If not managed well, they risk **emotional implosions** or anxiety-driven power struggles.

Strong Desire for Privacy and Control: Vulnerability can be challenging. Scorpio Rising tends to keep personal matters close to the chest and may test others' loyalty before opening up. They need to learn **healthy boundaries** without shutting people out.

Possible Reproductive or Elimination Concerns: As they rule these bodily systems, Scorpio Rising individuals should monitor sexual health, bladder/urinary care, and colon health (e.g., IBS or chronic inflammation). Emotional toxins can sometimes manifest in these areas.

Transformative Drive: Scorpio Rising people often crave deep change, whether psychological, spiritual, or material. They may gravitate toward healing professions, investigative fields, or areas that let them explore life's mysteries and transform hardships into strength.

Healing Potential and Resilience: The positive side of Scorpio's power is an **incredible ability to regenerate** after trauma. Scorpio Rising can harness this trait to heal themselves or guide others through crisis, reflecting the emotional intensity rooted in their prenatal origins.

Practical Guidance for Scorpio Rising Natives and Caregivers

Cultivating Emotional Awareness:
Journaling, therapy, or introspective arts can help Scorpio Rising process intense feelings without resorting to repression or secrecy.

Encouraging children to name and validate emotions fosters healthier coping and reduces the urge to hide vulnerabilities.

Supportive Environments for Trust-Building:
Scorpio Rising thrives in honest, loyal relationships. They benefit from consistent support—friends or mentors who respect their need for privacy but also gently encourage openness.

For children, stable home routines and clear communication about boundaries are crucial. Building trust early on helps them feel safe expressing deeper feelings.

Health Monitoring for Reproductive and Elimination Systems:

Regular checkups, balanced hydration, and a nutritious diet support the Scorpio-ruled organs.

Mindful detox strategies, like saunas, gentle cleanses, or stress-management techniques, can help prevent energy stagnation or toxic buildup.

Transformational Outlets:

Scorpio Rising individuals often need purposeful challenges, like intense study, investigative projects, or creative endeavors that channel their fervor constructively.

Engaging in martial arts or physically and mentally demanding activities can be a healthy expression of Mars/Pluto energy, fostering both discipline and emotional release.

Embracing Vulnerability as Strength:

Learning that genuine intimacy requires sharing fears and weaknesses is key.

Scorpio Rising's journey often involves redefining power, recognizing that courage to show softness can be transformational.

Encouraging deep and meaningful friendships or therapy can guide them toward letting go of destructive control patterns.

Conclusion

Scorpio Rising emerges from **potent gestational experiences** marked by deep emotional currents, potential secrecy, and a mother grappling with control or unresolved tension. These prenatal influences resonate with Scorpio's symbolic rulership of transformation, elimination, and emotional intensity. Modern scientific insights into maternal stress, epigenetics, and the power of suppressed or expressed emotions strongly parallel Scorpio's archetypal depth: the womb environment can indeed mold a child's capacity for suspicion, resilience, secrecy, and powerful emotional drives.

As adults, Scorpio Rising individuals possess a profound wellspring of intuition and regenerative potential, often guided by a passionate need to explore life's mysteries. Though they may wrestle with trust and control issues, they can also harness their intensity for tremendous personal growth, and, when directed positively, provide healing and insight for those around them. By cultivating honest self-awareness, balanced emotional expression, and healthy boundaries, Scorpio Rising natives honor their birthright of transformation, using it as a force for evolution rather than a constant personal battleground.

Chapter 9

Sagittarius Rising: Expansive Optimism and the Gestational Call to Adventure

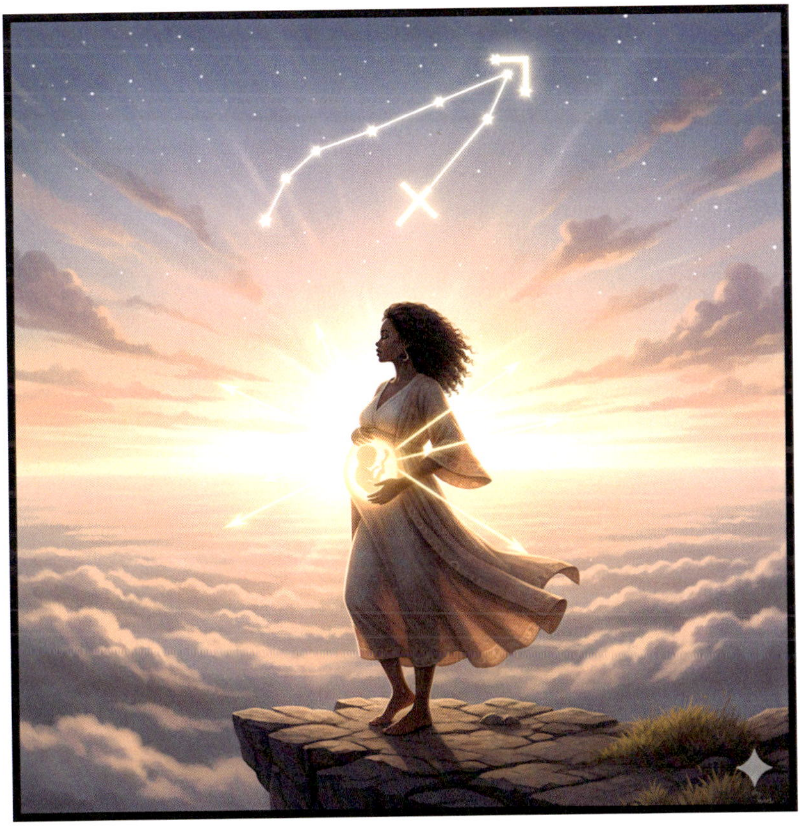

Introduction

Sagittarius is the ninth sign of the zodiac, traditionally ruled by Jupiter, symbolizing growth, faith, and a broadening of horizons. When Sagittarius appears on the Ascendant, individuals often embody a spirit of adventure, open-mindedness, and optimism—traits that may be shaped by the mother's pregnancy experiences. Medical astrologer Lynn Koiner's prenatal theory suggests that mothers of Sagittarius Rising children frequently report feeling physically and emotionally positive or encountering life changes that spur personal expansion. Such a gestational climate may prime the unborn child to expect opportunities and view life as an unfolding journey.

From a **medical astrology** perspective, Sagittarius is associated with the **hips, thighs, liver,** and the body's capacity for broad movement. Modern developmental research also illuminates how maternal well-being and confidence can foster resilience in the fetus, providing a parallel to Sagittarius Rising's trademark enthusiasm and openness.

In this chapter, we'll connect these threads, exploring how a prenatal sense of optimism and exploration can resonate throughout a Sagittarius Rising individual's life.

Sagittarius Rising in Traditional Medical Astrology
Classically, Sagittarius is linked to:

The Hips, Thighs, and Sciatic Nerve: Physically, Sagittarius Rising individuals may be prone to hip or thigh injuries if they overextend themselves in sports or travel.

The Liver and Metabolic Functions: Jupiter's influence can affect the body's assimilation and detoxification processes. An overabundance of indulgence might challenge liver health, mirroring Sagittarius' tendency to overdo things in pursuit of enjoyment.

Expansion, Vision, and Joy: Sagittarius Rising often exudes a **buoyant energy**, seeking knowledge, cultural experiences, or philosophical insights.

When balanced, this results in a naturally open-hearted and forward-looking personality.

Because Jupiter is often considered the "Great Benefic" in astrology, Sagittarius Ascendants can carry a sense of luck or protectedness. However, unchecked excess—whether in diet, travel, or risk-taking—can lead to health or lifestyle complications. Striking a balance between enthusiasm and moderation is a key lesson for Sagittarius Rising.

The Mother's Gestational Experience and Sagittarius Rising
Based on Lynn Koiner's observations, mothers of Sagittarius Rising babies often report:

Positive Physical Health and Emotional Uplift: Many felt particularly good during pregnancy—less morning sickness, more energy, and a general belief that "things are looking up." This environment of **optimism** can imprint the fetus with an innate orientation toward faith and possibility.

A Sense of Expansion or New Horizons: Some mothers experienced a major move, a new job, or even spiritual awakenings (engaging with new philosophies or religious beliefs). The unborn child may thus "learn" the importance of exploration and open-mindedness.

Hope-Filled Mindset and Future-Focused Attitudes: In several anecdotes, mothers described being filled with hope and anticipation, often placing strong faith in better circumstances just around the corner. This resonates with Sagittarius Rising's confidence and adventurous orientation in adulthood.

Encounters with Cultural or Educational Opportunities: Because Sagittarius thrives on learning, mothers might have embarked on classes, travel, or cross-cultural experiences during pregnancy. The child can inherit these "broadening" influences, fueling a lifelong interest in higher knowledge and diverse perspectives.

Modern Prenatal Research: Biological Underpinnings
Contemporary science supports the notion that a mother's positive emotional state and sense of possibility can tangibly impact fetal development:

Maternal Positivity and Stress Regulation:

Mothers who experience steady optimism or an "upward mood trajectory" generally produce less cortisol and more feel-good hormones (like dopamine or endorphins). This stable biochemical environment fosters a resilient fetal HPA axis, potentially leading to a child who can bounce back from stress.

Babies of mothers who feel a sense of hope or faith during pregnancy often demonstrate adaptive coping and a natural inclination toward curiosity, paralleling Sagittarius Rising's openness.

Movement and Physical Activity:

If the mother's expansion includes physical mobility, exercise, exploration, or travel, studies show it can improve cardiovascular health, leading to better-oxygenated fetal development.

A mother's regular physical activity can prime the child for a robust constitution, reflecting Sagittarius' inclination toward movement and athleticism.

Cultural and Educational Exposure:

Prenatal periods filled with learning, be it language acquisition, reading, or exposure to varied cultural stimuli, can support the fetus's early neurological development. The child may show a natural curiosity later in life, akin to Sagittarius Rising's wanderlust for knowledge.

Cross-cultural or intellectual influences may shape a fetus's emerging sense of "normal," leaving them more receptive to new or global perspectives, a core Sagittarian trait.

Faith and Future-Focused Mindset:

Psychological studies suggest that maternal hopefulness can lower anxiety and reduce the chances of perinatal depression. Lower maternal depression correlates with better emotional outcomes in infancy, supporting a child's positive worldview.

Sagittarius Rising's characteristic confidence and philosophical bend might echo these prenatal underpinnings of trust in a brighter future.

Sagittarius Rising in Adulthood:

Health and Emotional PatternsWhen they reach adulthood, Sagittarius Rising individuals often:

Embrace a Broad Life Perspective:

They're attracted to **travel, education, and cultural exchanges**, seeking constant growth and new experiences. Stagnation or narrow thinking typically frustrates them.

Exude Optimism and Risk-Taking Behaviors: Faith in a positive outcome can lead them to leap into opportunities, but it may also tempt them to overextend—physically, financially, or socially.

Experience Potential Hip, Thigh, or Liver Strains: A high-energy lifestyle, indulgent eating or drinking, and a love of "adventure sports" can put stress on their Sagittarian regions (hips, thighs) and overburden the liver if moderation is not practiced.

Seek Ethical or Philosophical Frameworks: Sagittarius Rising might gravitate toward **religion, spirituality, or philosophical pursuits**. They're often motivated by the quest for meaning beyond immediate gratification.

Possess Natural Resilience:
Many bounce back from setbacks with encouraging self talk, a trait that likely originated in the supportive or uplifting prenatal environment their mothers described.

Practical Guidance for Sagittarius Rising Natives and Caregivers

Encourage Healthy Exploration:

Travel, sports, and intellectual endeavors suit Sagittarius Rising's appetite for newness. However, guide them to plan or research sufficiently to avoid reckless risks.

Activities that blend **physical movement and learning** (like cultural dance classes, nature treks with educational components) can nurture body and mind simultaneously.

Mindful Moderation:

Teach them early about portion control—both in diet and in life pursuits, so that Jupiter's love of abundance doesn't lead to overindulgence.

Adults can benefit from detox or balanced eating protocols, paying special attention to liver health and ensuring adequate rest between bouts of high-intensity living.

Channel Optimism into Realistic Goals:

While positivity fuels ambition, setting achievable milestones prevents frustration. Sagittarius Rising thrives with supportive structures that let them dream big while staying grounded.

Emphasize goal-planning skills and time management, so that broad visions don't get lost in daily distractions.

Harness Their Philosophical Drive:

Spiritual or ethical frameworks can direct their innate curiosity and moral compass. Encouraging them to study various belief systems expands their worldview while aligning with Sagittarian idealism.

Group activities like book clubs, philosophical salons, or volunteering offer social engagement, knowledge exchange, and a sense of mission.

Foster Emotional Responsibility:

Teach children to handle disappointment or obstacles constructively, without glossing over real problems.

True resilience comes from acknowledging challenges, then forging ahead with pragmatic hope.

Adults might consider meditation or mindfulness to temper restlessness, bridging their big-picture optimism with daily emotional steadiness.

Conclusion

Sagittarius Rising emerges from a prenatal environment marked by **expansion, optimism, and a mother's faith in better horizons**. Under these conditions, the fetus may absorb a worldview steeped in hope, mobility, and openness hallmarks of Jupiter's influence. Contemporary research underscores how a mother's buoyant mood, dynamic physical activities, and cultural or educational pursuits can shape a child's resilience, curiosity, and positive affect.

In adulthood, Sagittarius Rising individuals often serve as enthusiastic explorers whether in travel, academia, or philosophical inquiry.

Their high-energy approach, when balanced by thoughtful moderation and emotional responsibility, can lead to remarkable achievements and uplifting leadership. By recognizing the prenatal roots of their adventurous spirit, Sagittarius Rising natives can more deliberately harness their Jupiterian gifts, transforming raw optimism into a meaningful life path of growth, discovery, and shared inspiration.

Chapter 10

Capricorn Rising: Enduring Determination and the Weight of Responsibility in the Womb

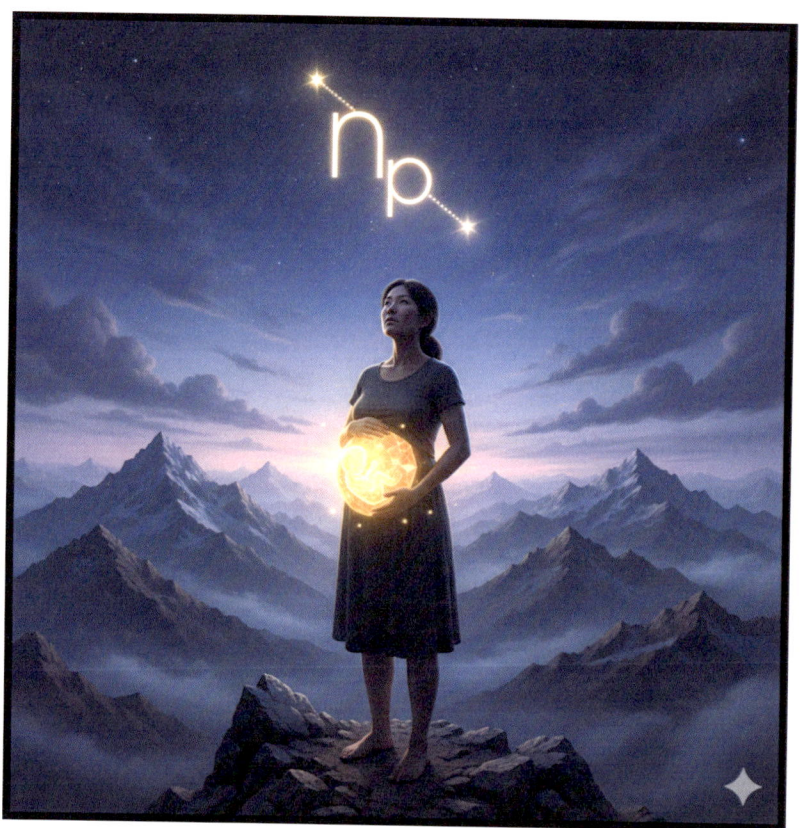

Introduction

Capricorn, the tenth sign of the zodiac, is traditionally ruled by Saturn, symbolizing structure, responsibility, and the lessons of time. When Capricorn appears on the Ascendant, individuals often exude a reserved, cautious, and determined demeanor. According to medical astrologer Lynn Koiner's prenatal theory, these Capricornian qualities may have roots in the mother's emotional experiences during pregnancy—particularly if she felt a sense of dread, anxiety, or the weight of obligations.

From a medical astrology standpoint, Capricorn is associated with the bones (especially the knees), skin, joints, and the body's structural integrity. Modern prenatal research on maternal stress, worry, and mood parallels this sign's themes: the fetus may absorb a sense of seriousness or guardedness if the mother grapples with uncertainty or impending responsibilities. Together, these views shed light on how Capricorn Rising embodies a steady, self-reliant disposition that can be both a source of strength and a channel for cautious reserve.

119

Capricorn Rising in Traditional Medical Astrology
Classically, Capricorn and Saturn rule over:

Bones, Joints, and Skeletal System: Capricorn Rising individuals are often physically sturdy but may experience joint stiffness (especially knee problems) or skin issues when under prolonged stress.

A Sense of Constraint and Responsibility: Saturn's influence instills discipline and structure; however, it can also manifest as rigidity or anxiety around duties.

Slow but Steady Growth: Capricorn Ascendants tend to mature early and adopt a serious outlook on life. They typically reach greater ease or success later in life, aligning with Saturn's reputation as a late-blooming but long-lasting energy.

Because Capricorn is an earth sign, it emphasizes practicality and realism. Yet, with Saturn's weight, a Capricorn Rising can incline toward caution, self-containment, and guardedness—traits that may connect directly to the mother's prenatal emotional state.

The Mother's Gestational Experience and Capricorn Rising

Lynn Koiner's findings suggest that mothers of Capricorn Rising children often experienced:

Anxiety or Dread about the Pregnancy: This can occur if the child was the first or the last in the family. With a firstborn, the mother may have worried about her new responsibilities; with a lastborn, she might have felt certain this "had to be the final one" and felt ambivalence or pressure, especially if the pregnancy was unplanned.

Fear of External Pressures: In some cases, the mother worried about finances, housing, or the demands of in-laws. Such looming obligations often parallel Capricorn's internal sense of carrying burdens.

Emotional Reserve or Preoccupation: The mother might not have openly displayed negativity but instead held a subdued or solemn outlook ("I must soldier on"). This stoicism can imprint the fetus with an internalized expectation of self-reliance.

Seriousness and Duty: Even if the mother wanted the child, she could have faced heavy responsibilities or a work situation that reduced her joy. The unborn child might interpret these signals as "the world is serious—prepare accordingly," fitting Capricorn's cautious mindset.

ModernPrenatal Research: Biological Underpinnings Current scientific studies highlight mechanisms by which maternal anxiety, dread, or over-responsibility can shape fetal development:

Chronic Stress and HPA Axis Calibration:

Long-term worry or dread elevates cortisol in the mother, which can pass through the placenta. Babies exposed to persistent cortisol may emerge with a heightened baseline for stress and a predisposition toward vigilance or anxious caution.

Such children might show early maturity (behaving "older than their years") as a survival strategy, resonating with Capricorn Rising's serious disposition.

Maternal Mood and Infant Temperament:

Research on maternal depression or consistent worry indicates that these emotional states can dampen or slow a child's early sense of spontaneity, causing them to appear more inhibited. This can parallel the Capricorn Rising's reserved approach.

If the mother also provided stable routines despite her worry, the child might gain a sense of reliability in structure—a hallmark of Capricorn's methodical nature.

Bone and Skeletal Development:

While direct scientific correlations between maternal stress and fetal bone development are ongoing, stress-related hormonal imbalances can affect overall fetal growth. A stable regimen of prenatal vitamins and consistent checkups might mitigate these effects.

Astrologically, strong Saturn vibes might symbolize the baby "building a firm backbone" in response to maternal uncertainty, though biologically the connection is less direct.

Early Responsibility and Self-Sufficiency:

Some studies suggest that children who sense maternal stress might try to "adapt" in the womb, potentially leading to heightened self-regulatory skills later. Capricorn Rising's independent streak could reflect such prenatal responsibility conditioning.

Capricorn Rising in Adulthood: Health and Emotional Patterns

By adulthood, Capricorn Rising individuals often exhibit:

Stoicism and Reserve: They may come across as cool or distant initially, trusting others only after observing consistent reliability.

Early Maturity or a "Serious" Demeanor: Capricorn Rising people frequently feel compelled to prove themselves, sometimes carrying an internal sense of having to work harder than everyone else.

Skeletal and Skin Watchpoints: Knees, joints, teeth, and skin can be vulnerable under prolonged stress (e.g.,

ension-related issues like eczema or arthritic flare-ups). Regular care of these areas is important.

Ambition and Enduring Work Ethic: Over time, Capricorn Rising individuals can achieve recognition through persistent effort. They do well with long-term goals and step-by-step progress.

Difficulty Accepting Support: Because they learned (even prenatally) that the world can be burdensome, they may be reluctant to ask for help or share responsibilities. This can lead to stress accumulation if not addressed.

Practical Guidance for Capricorn Rising Natives and Caregivers
Nurture Emotional Expression:
Encourage Capricorn Rising children to voice worries or insecurities rather than internalizing them. This helps alleviate the pressure to appear endlessly self-sufficient.

Adult Capricorn Risings may benefit from journaling, therapy, or group activities that gently challenge their,

reserve.

Balanced Ambition and Self-Care:

Setting **realistic goals** rather than overwhelming ones ensures progress without burnout. Breaking major tasks into smaller, doable steps suits their methodical approach.

Incorporate **stress-reduction techniques** (mindful breathing, massages, gentle stretching) that specifically target the joints, spine, and back.

Encourage Patience and Self-Compassion:
Capricorn Rising can be tough on themselves, feeling that everything rests on their shoulders. Validation and acceptance of small wins can build confidence over time.

Teach them it's okay to lean on others—delegating or collaborating can lighten the burden of perpetual self-reliance.

Support Skeletal Health:

Calcium-rich foods, weight-bearing exercises, and maintaining good posture help prevent knee or back issues.

Keeping an eye on stress levels is key: chronic tension can manifest in joint stiffness or skin breakouts.

Long-Term Planning with Flexibility:
While Capricorn thrives on planning and structure, life can throw curveballs. Encouraging them to stay open to changes fosters resilience.

Celebrating incremental achievements helps them avoid discouragement when aiming for big, Saturn-like milestones.

Conclusion

Capricorn Rising emerges from a prenatal environment deeply influenced by anxiety, burden, or a sense of dread surrounding the pregnancy. In such conditions, the fetus may internalize signals that caution,

self-containment, and preparation for hard work are essential strategies for survival—perfectly aligned with Saturn's imprint. Modern research on maternal stress confirms that babies can indeed adapt their stress responses to reflect the mother's emotional milieu, potentially leading to the seriousness and self-reliance observed in Capricorn Rising.

In adulthood, Capricorn Rising individuals are known for tenacity, maturity, and resilience, but they must also watch out for chronic stress manifested in skeletal tension or emotional reserve. By acknowledging the possible gestational roots of their cautious outlook, Capricorn Rising natives can harness Saturn's gifts endurance, responsibility, and wisdom without becoming weighed down by internalized burdens. Through balanced ambition, genuine self-care, and the willingness to seek support, they transform early imprints of dread into a dignified path of steady achievement.

Chapter 11

Aquarius Rising: Rebellion, Independence, and the Womb's Urge for Freedom

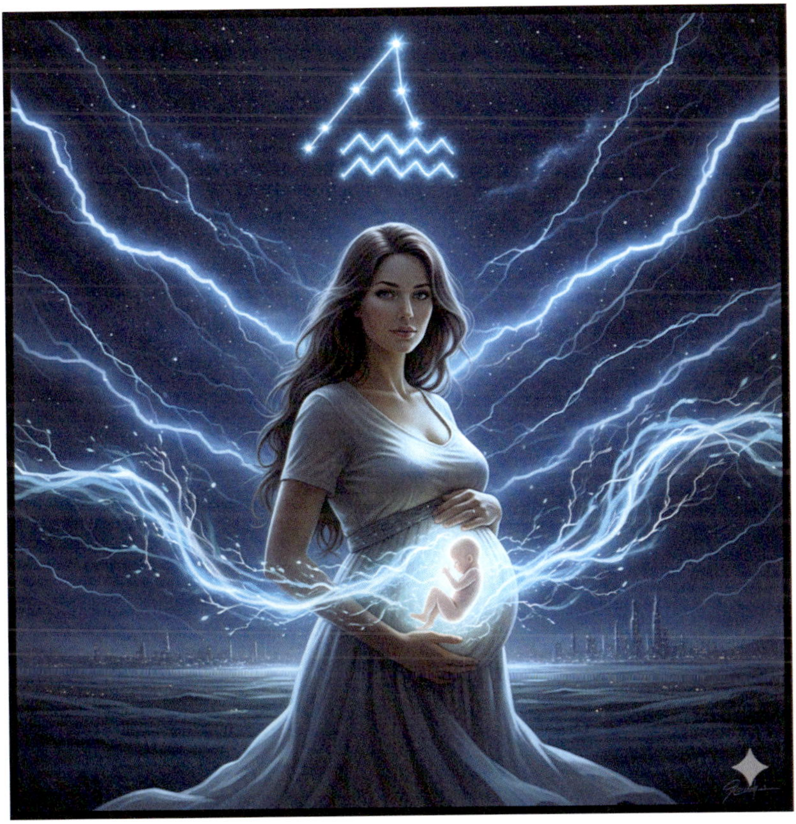

Introduction

Aquarius is the eleventh sign of the zodiac, traditionally ruled by Saturn and, in modern astrology, by Uranus. It symbolizes innovation, individuality, and a progressive view of society. When Aquarius appears on the Ascendant, individuals often grow into self-reliant, open-minded, and sometimes contrarian personalities—traits that, according to medical astrologer Lynn Koiner's prenatal theory, may trace back to the mother's psychological or social environment during pregnancy.

Medical astrology connects Aquarius with the circulatory system, the ankles, and electrical or nerve impulses in the body, reflecting this sign's dynamic, quick-moving qualities. Modern prenatal research resonates with the idea that a mother's rebellious attitudes, sudden lifestyle changes, or desire for autonomy can imprint on the fetus, cultivating a comfort with unpredictability, forward-thinking ideals, and a "question everything" mentality. This chapter explores how these influences shape Aquarius Rising's hallmark traits of independence and ingenuity.

Aquarius Rising in Traditional Medical Astrology

Classically, Aquarius is linked to:

Circulation, Blood, and Lower Legs (Ankles): Aquarius Rising individuals may be sensitive to circulation issues, cramps in the calves and ankles, or general nerve-related stresses.

Electrical Energies and Nervous System: In modern interpretation, Uranus is associated with rapid, "electric" impulses, reflecting the sudden insights or eccentricities of Aquarius. Nervous agitation or restlessness can arise if life feels too restrictive.

Collective Ideals and Detachment: Aquarius often seeks freedom from tradition, placing emphasis on innovative, humanitarian, or egalitarian concerns. On the Ascendant, it fosters a socially aware but sometimes emotionally detached presentation.

131

While Saturn's old rulership of Aquarius brings structure and intellect, Uranus adds a spark of rebellion and unpredictability. Balancing these forces can lead Aquarius Rising to be both pragmatically mindful and creatively disruptive in equal measure.

The Mother's Gestational Experience and Aquarius Rising
Drawing from Lynn Koiner's observations:

Rebellion or Desire for Autonomy: Mothers of Aquarius Rising children often report feeling the need to "break away" from family expectations, medical advice, or rigid social norms. They might have insisted on their own birth plan despite doctors' warnings, or bucked tradition in some other aspect of pregnancy.

Unexpected Shifts and Challenges: Some mothers faced sudden changes—job relocations, health concerns, or relationship upheavals. This unpredictability may translate into the child's eventual comfort with rapid change.

Refusal to Conform: A mother's rebellious streak—however mild—can form a prenatal message of "forge your own path, question authority." The unborn child often soaks up these signals, later manifesting as independent thinking and a quirkiness that sets Aquarius Rising apart.

Social-Change Mindset: In some cases, the mother became involved with advocacy or social movements during pregnancy, channeling a sense of collective betterment. The fetus may come into the world primed for activism, progressive ideas, or championing group causes.

Modern Prenatal Research: Biological Underpinnings
Contemporary science offers insights on how rebellious attitudes, sudden life shifts, and maternal stress can shape fetal development:

Maternal Autonomy and Cortisol Regulation:
When a mother resists authority or external pressure—sometimes in an act of empowerment—she may feel,

bursts of adrenaline and cortisol that come with standing her ground.

In moderate amounts, these hormones can galvanize a fetus's stress response system, potentially fostering resilience and a heightened capacity to handle sudden changes—mirroring Aquarius's adaptability.

Epigenetics and Radical Shifts:

Dramatic changes or sudden moves can alter maternal hormone balances, immune responses, and daily routines. Epigenetic studies suggest that repeated disruptions to a mother's environment can prime the fetus for **flexibility**—both biologically and psychologically.

This aligns with Aquarius Rising's aptitude for quick adaptation and comfort in unconventional settings.

Social Consciousness and Oxytocin Pathways:

Maternal involvement in community projects or activism,

may raise oxytocin levels and feelings of social connectedness. Babies exposed to consistent maternal social engagement might develop an other-oriented perspective—a hallmark of Aquarius's humanitarian leanings.

Conversely, if the mother is rebellious in isolation—fueling anger at societal structures—this might orient the fetus toward distrust of authority, another signature of Aquarius Rising.

Nervous System Sensitivity:

Sudden events and unpredictability can stimulate the mother's sympathetic nervous system. If the mother copes positively, it can boost healthy stress management in the fetus. If not, the fetus may internalize a more erratic or anxious response—Aquarius Rising can manifest as restlessness or mental hyperactivity.

Such influences underscore the need for consistent emotional support even amid rebellious or unconventional pregnancy choices.

Aquarius Rising in Adulthood: Health and Emotional Patterns

As adults, Aquarius Rising individuals often display:

Independent and Innovative Thinking: They're attracted to original ideas, new technology, or radical social theories. They prefer forging their own route rather than conforming to established norms.

Social Awareness Coupled with Emotional Detachment: They excel at seeing the "big picture" of group dynamics but may struggle with overt displays of sentiment, sometimes appearing cool or aloof.

Rebellion Against Restriction: Attempts to confine their behavior often trigger resistance. They value freedom, autonomy, and the right to define life on their own terms.

Potential Circulatory Vulnerabilities: Varicose veins, ankle sprains, or foot/leg cramps may arise under,

stress or inactivity. Keeping circulation strong via regular movement is key.

Spike-and-Drop Energy Patterns: True to Uranus's sudden bursts, Aquarius Rising folks can surge with enthusiasm for a cause or project, then abruptly pivot when boredom strikes—learning to channel this effectively is vital for long-term success.

Practical Guidance for Aquarius Rising Natives and Caregivers

Embrace Individuality While Encouraging Connection:

Aquarius Rising children benefit from understanding **shared humanity**. Balance personal freedoms with empathy-building activities (team sports, volunteer projects) that promote collaboration.

For adults, consciously practicing emotional vulnerability can stave off excessive detachment.

137

Support Circulatory Health:

Integrate regular exercise—especially those stimulating the lower legs (e.g., walking, cycling)—to improve blood flow.

Avoid extended periods of sitting; get up and stretch often. Techniques like cold-water therapy or massages might help keep circulation optimized.

Structured Flexibility:

Provide guidelines rather than rigid rules. Aquarius Rising typically rejects overly strict authority but can thrive with open-ended structures.

Encourage them to experiment within boundaries—like free-form projects or the choice to lead personal initiatives.

Focus on Meaningful Innovation:

Channel rebellious urges into creative or humanitarian solutions. Whether it's coding a new app, spearheading community efforts, or pioneering environmental,

movements, Aquarius Rising is motivated by progress.

For children, highlight the "why" behind rules or lessons, inviting them to suggest improvements.

Techno and Community Balance:

Aquarius Rising often loves technology but should also engage in face-to-face relationships and nature-based activities to prevent social or emotional detachment.

Managing screen time—especially for kids—and cultivating real-world ties fosters a healthy balance between futuristic thinking and grounded human connection.

Conclusion

Aquarius Rising emerges from a prenatal environment that features rebelliousness, sudden changes, or strong drives for personal autonomy. These maternal experiences often encode a spirit of progress,

independence, and adaptability in the fetus. Modern research on maternal stress responses, epigenetics, and social engagement supports the idea that a child can be biologically and psychologically primed to challenge norms and remain comfortable with change.

As adults, Aquarius Rising individuals frequently excel as inventors, reformers, or visionaries in their fields. They prize freedom and originality, but they must also guard against emotional distance and restlessness.

By acknowledging the gestational roots of their contrarian bent, Aquarius Rising natives can channel their innate rebellious streak into purposeful innovation and humane activism. Embracing both autonomy and genuine connection allows them to fulfill the promise of their cosmic blueprint serving the collective good while staying authentically themselves.

Chapter 12

Pisces Rising: Empathy, Creativity, and the Womb's "Tuned-Out" Vibration

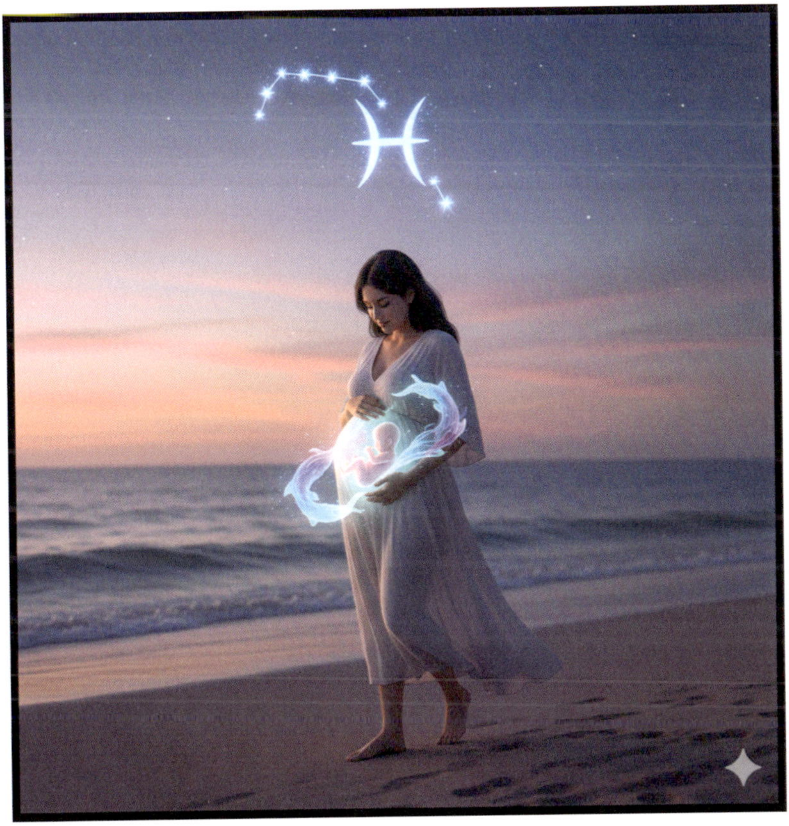

Introduction

Pisces is the twelfth sign of the zodiac, traditionally ruled by Jupiter and in modern astrology often associated with Neptune. It symbolizes empathy, imagination, and a fluid sense of identity. When Pisces appears on the Ascendant, individuals may display profound sensitivity and a pronounced intuitive streak—traits that, according to medical astrologer Lynn Koiner's prenatal theory, can be traced back to the mother's emotional landscape during pregnancy.

Medical astrology links Pisces with the **feet, lymphatic system, and the body's overall fluid balance**, emphasizing a keen receptivity to environmental cues. Modern prenatal studies further suggest that maternal Pisces Rising in Traditional Medical Astrology

Pisces is classically associated with:

Feet and the Lymphatic System: Pisces Rising individuals may experience foot sensitivity, water retention, or swelling if balance is disrupted. They often benefit from grounding practices that address fluid circulation.

Mysticism and Imagination: Often deemed the most sensitive sign, Pisces can inspire compassion, spirituality, and deep creative gifts—but also an inclination toward escapism or dependency if not channeled productively.

Empathic Boundaries: As a mutable water sign, Pisces Rising is exceptionally open to external energies, often needing to develop, strong emotional and psychic boundaries to maintain well-being.

The hallmark of Pisces Rising is permeability, the ability to soak in impressions from their environment, just as fish absorb the qualities of the water they swim in. This heightened openness is a double-edged sword, fueling compassion and creativity yet leaving them prone to overwhelm.

The Mother's Gestational Experience and Pisces Rising
In Lynn Koiner's research, mothers of Pisces Rising children frequently reported:

Tuning Out or Escapism: Some mothers felt ,

emotionally distant or ambivalent about the pregnancy. Others coped with stress through art, daydreaming, or even substance use. This sense of "not being fully there" may imprint the fetus with a fluid, less-grounded sense of reality.

Heightened Sensitivity or Vulnerability: If the mother was fearful, in ill health, or dealing with complex life situations, she might have sought emotional numbing. The child, meanwhile, absorbs unresolved anxieties and a subconscious desire to escape difficulties.

Creative and Spiritual Immersion: On a positive note, mothers who turned to music, painting, or spiritual practices (meditation, prayer, mysticism) during pregnancy often noted a calmer sense of detachment. The fetus may then develop strong intuitive or artistic leanings, hallmarks of Pisces' inspirational energy.

Ambivalent Emotions: Mothers who were unsure about having another child or who faced conflicting life choices might have oscillated between warmth and

disinterest. This could produce a child uncertain about where they truly belong, reflecting Pisces Rising's sometimes elusive self-image.

Modern Prenatal Research: Biological Underpinnings
Contemporary science provides context for how maternal escapism or creative engagement can affect fetal development:

Maternal Stress and Avoidance Behaviors:

Chronic stress can drive a pregnant mother to disengage or "tune out." Elevated cortisol levels may be partially masked by coping strategies (ranging from creative outlets to substances like alcohol or medication).

If the mother feels disconnected, the fetus may be exposed to inconsistent emotional or hormonal signals, leading to a child who can be highly empathic yet unsure of how to ground themselves.

Neurological Sensitivity and Dopamine Pathways:

Creative activities and fantasy can raise dopamine levels, which might buffer some negative stress effects. The fetus could inherit a heightened openness to imaginative realms.

However, inconsistent or extreme maternal mood states can imprint the fetal brain with fluctuating stress responses, aligning with Pisces Rising's mutable, ever-shifting disposition.

Substance Use or Medication:

n some instances, the mother might resort to sedatives, painkillers, or other substances that induce a dreamy or numbed state. This can alter fetal neural development, possibly creating heightened sensitivity or predisposition to addictive behaviors later.

Modern research underscores the risks of prenatal exposure to substances; astrologically, it resonates with Pisces Rising's potential struggles around escapism or emotional boundaries.

Ambivalence and Epigenetics:

Epigenetic studies show that maternal ambivalence or strong emotional swings can affect how genes regulating stress and mood expression are activated in the fetus.

For Pisces Rising, this may result in a predisposition toward deep empathy, subtle emotional fluctuations, and an urge to blend with (or escape from) their surroundings.

Pisces Rising in Adulthood: Health and Emotional Patterns

As adults, Pisces Rising individuals typically exhibit:

High Empathy and Sensitivity: They often pick up on others' emotions easily and can be deeply compassionate. Over time, they may need to learn discernment to avoid absorbing too much negativity.

Artistic or Spiritual Inclinations: Pisces Rising people frequently feel at home in music, dance, film,

147

metaphysics, or any realm that honors dreams and imagination. These outlets can be profoundly healing when used constructively.

Struggles with Boundaries: Their fluid nature can invite confusing or codependent relationships if they don't establish healthy emotional parameters. They may also retreat into fantasy or addictive behaviors under extreme stress.

Susceptibility to Overwhelm: Because they're so permeable, hectic environments or excessive demands can lead to fatigue, anxiety, and the urge to withdraw. They thrive in tranquil spaces.

Physical Manifestations: Foot issues, edema, or psychosomatic symptoms can flare up when emotional stress isn't addressed. Pisces Rising might also be more receptive to holistic therapies that engage the mind-body-spirit connection.

Practical Guidance for Pisces Rising Natives and

Caregivers

Establish Clear Emotional Boundaries:
Teach children (and remind adults) how to differentiate their feelings from others', practices like journaling, guided visualizations, or mindful breathing can help.

Encourage them to say "no" when necessary, fostering a healthy sense of self within their empathy for others.

o

Channel Creativity and Spirituality:

Pisces Rising individuals thrive on artistic expression, painting, music, dance, poetry, and often find solace in spiritual or meditative practices. These pathways provide safe emotional release.

Cultivating daily rituals (like lighting a candle, practicing yoga, or journaling) helps them remain grounded while navigating their intuitive depths.

Balance Escapism with Real-World Engagement:

Provide gentle structure—schedules, reminders, or supportive guidance—so they can handle practical tasks without feeling pinned down.

If escapist tendencies are strong, encourage healthy escapes such as imaginative storytelling, nature walks, or creative hobbies rather than substance use or perpetual daydreaming.

Mindful Physical Care:

Activities like swimming, foot massage, reflexology, and gentle stretching (yin yoga) can be especially beneficial for Pisces Rising, supporting both the feet and fluid circulation.

Emotional tension often reflects in their body. Regular relaxation baths, breathwork, or floating tanks can soothe heightened nervous energy.

Cultivate Safe Havens:

Having a **calm, nurturing environment** (color palettes, soft music, a personal sanctuary) helps them

recharge.

Socially, they do best with a few trustworthy confidants who respect their sensitivity. Support from empathetic mentors or friends can keep them from feeling lost in chaotic social settings.

Conclusion

Pisces Rising emerges from a prenatal environment in which the mother's emotional or mental presence was often fragmented, escapist, or creatively immersive. These womb conditions may teach the fetus that reality is fluid and boundaries can be indistinct—mirroring Pisces' mutable, watery nature. Modern research affirms that maternal ambivalence, artistic pursuits, or substance use can significantly influence the child's neurological wiring, predisposing them to heightened empathy, imagination, and occasional struggles with grounding.

As adults, Pisces Rising individuals embody a mystical, deeply compassionate energy that can foster profound

creativity and healing abilities. Yet they also need strong boundaries and self-care routines to avoid the pitfalls of escapism, codependence, or emotional overwhelm. By honoring the dreamy seeds planted in utero and consciously learning to navigate their empathic gifts, Pisces Rising natives can transform their prenatal legacy into a life of boundless inspiration, meaningful service, and spiritual wisdom.

References

Astrological and Medical Astrology Sources

Koiner, Lynn. Gestation and the Ascendant: The Mother's Role in the Development of the Rising Sign. [Unpublished notes and lectures, 2000–2020]. Available at: www.lynnkoiner.com

Hill, Judith. Medical Astrology: A Guide to Planetary Pathology. Portland, OR: Stellium Press, 2004.

Lehman, Lee. Classical Medical Astrology: Healing with the Elements. Whitford Press, 2019.

Cornell, Howard L. Encyclopedia of Medical Astrology. Astrology Classics, 2003 (original 1933).

Culpeper, Nicholas. Culpeper's Complete Herbal. London, 1653.

Hadzic, Eileen Nauman. Medical Astrology for Healing. Blue Turtle Publishing, 2002.

References

Scientific and Psychological References

Van den Bergh, B. R. H., et al. (2005). Antenatal maternal anxiety and stress and the neurobehavioral development of the fetus and child: links and possible mechanisms. Neuroscience & Biobehavioral Reviews, 29(2), 237–258.

DiPietro, J. A. (2010). Psychological and psychophysiological considerations regarding the maternal–fetal relationship. Infant and Child Development, 19(1), 27–38.

Glover, V. (2014). *Maternal depression, anxiety and stress during pregnancy and child outcome; what needs to be done.* Best Practice & Research Clinical Obstetrics & Gynaecology, 28(1), 25–35.

Monk, C., Lugo-Candelas, C., & Trumpff, C. (2019). Prenatal developmental origins of future psychopathology: mechanisms and pathways. Annual Review of Clinical Psychology, 15, 317–344.

References

Yehuda, R., & Bierer, L. M. (2009). *The relevance of epigenetics to PTSD: implications for the DSM-V.* Journal of Traumatic Stress, 22(5), 427–434.

Lester, B. M., & Padbury, J. F. (2009). *Third pathophysiology of prenatal stress: the developmental impact of stress and adversity on neurobehavioral outcomes.* Early Human Development, 85(11), 737–741.

Additional Resources for Cross-Referencing

Pert, Candace. Molecules of Emotion: Why You Feel the Way You Feel. Scribner, 1997.

Verny, Thomas, & Kelly, John. The Secret Life of the Unborn Child. Dell Publishing, 1981.
Chamberlain, David B. Windows to the Womb: Revealing the Conscious Baby from Conception to Birth. North Atlantic Books, 2013.

References

Bruce Lipton, Ph.D. The Biology of Belief: Unleashing the Power of Consciousness, Matter & Miracles. Hay House, 2005.

Odent, Michel. The Scientification of Love. Free Association Books, 2001.

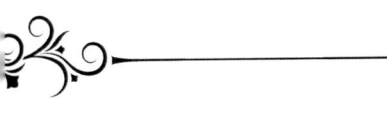

About the Book

Before the First Breath: The Womb's Imprint on the Rising Sign and Personality

Who were you before you were born?

In this eye-opening book, Cynthia Reneé Sumpter reveals that your Rising Sign, the Ascendant, is more than just the mask you wear. It's the first imprint of your life, shaped in the womb by your mother's emotions, health, and daily experiences.

Blending astrology, prenatal psychology, and modern science, Before the First Breath uncovers how each Ascendant reflects a gestational story. The fiery rush of Aries, the calm grounding of Taurus, the sensitivity of Cancer, the radiant glow of Leo, each Rising Sign mirrors the environment your mother carried you in.

Through vivid explanations and practical insights, you'll learn how the womb experience influences personality, resilience, and even health patterns later in life. More importantly, you'll discover how awareness of these prenatal imprints can guide healing, self-understanding, and transformation.

Whether you're an astrologer, a parent, or simply curious about your cosmic beginnings, this book offers a new way to see your Rising Sign, not just as destiny, but as the echo of your very first home: the womb.

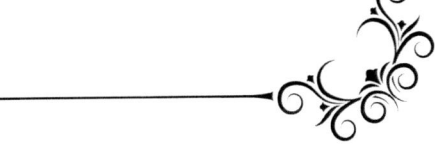